"Pope Brock reaches into the past and captures an
incredible story . . . perceptive."

—*Chicago Sun-Times*

"Written with glee, in a style that is pure gusto, a bubbling fountain
of metaphor and arresting image . . . Fishbein's campaign against
Brinkley makes up one strand of this extraordinary tale and provides
it with a bravura courtroom finale."

—*Boston Globe*

"Hugely amusing [but also] dark and cautionary, a reminder of the high
price of gullibility and ignorance."

—Jonathan Yardley, *Washington Post Book World*

"With a mix of down-home charm and breathless storytelling,
CHARLATAN makes for a compelling slice of lurid Americana . . .
fun to read."

—*Entertainment Weekly*

"Fascinating . . . Brock is gifted."

—*Associated Press*

"Brock captures the shamelessness and adaptability that make
Brinkley fascinating."

—*The New Yorker*

"Stunning . . . [*CHARLATAN*] chronicles, with a rollicking sense of fun
mixed with outrage, the truly unbelievable career of Brinkley."

—*Atlanta Journal-Constitution*

"Excellent . . . contains an implicit warning for our own age
of quick-fix quacks."

—*Times Literary Supplement*

"Pope Brock's true-life account of this comic-evil monster is nothing less
than Twainian: a blend of reportage, social history, portraiture, and
storytelling in the gland—excuse me, in the grand—tradition."

—Ron Powers, author of *Mark Twain: A Life*
and coauthor of *Flags of Our Fathers*

"If Hollywood hasn't already optioned [this], what's keeping it?"
—David Gates, *Newsweek*

"Stranger than fiction doesn't really say it. This is a book you won't put down and a story you'll never forget."
—James R. Gaines, author of *For Liberty and Glory: Washington, Lafayette, and Their Revolutions*

"**This spellbinding saga of a once-famous medical man who left all too many corpses in his wake is nothing short of spectacular.** Impeccably researched, smartly crafted, beautifully written, it's a pure joy to read. And dealing, as it does, with eternal traits of human greed and gullibility, this extraordinary book is timely as well as timeless . . . A mesmerizing must-read, written by a writer of exquisite talent . . . **One is left with the kind of reaction one has after reading a masterpiece.**"
—Heinz Kohler, Willard Long Thorp Professor of Economics Emeritus, Amherst College

"With sprightly style, Brock exposes the randy rise of a master huckster and his fall at the hands of a relentless quack hunter. It's a fine account of medical fakery, congenital scientific stupidity, and the habitual human appetite for being fooled and exploited . . . **Wonderful American social history and lots of fun.**"
—*Kirkus Reviews*

"**Rollicking, funny, brilliantly readable.**"
—*Mail on Sunday (London Daily Mail)*

"An irresistible and wide-ranging slice of popular history . . . lively and fascinating."
—*Seattle Times*

"**Shocking and hilarious in equal measure** . . . a cautionary tale for our own times—about celebrity, mass-marketing, media power, political huckstering, and the dangerous allure of mumbo-jumbo. **As irresistible as Brinkley's snake oil, and far more invigorating, *CHARLATAN* is an instant classic.**"
—Francis Wheen, author of *How Mumbo-Jumbo Conquered the World* and *The Irresistible Con: The Bizarre Life of a Fraudulent Genius*

Charlatan

America's Most Dangerous Huckster,

the Man Who Pursued Him,

and the Age of Flimflam

Pope Brock

THREE RIVERS PRESS • NEW YORK

Three Rivers Press and the Tugboat design are registered
trademarks of Random House, Inc.

Originally published in hardcover in the United States by
Crown Publishers, an imprint of the Crown Publishing Group, a division of
Random House, Inc., New York, in 2008.

Grateful acknowledgment is made to the following for permission to reprint
previously published material:

Peer International Corporation: Excerpt from "I'm Thinking Tonight of My Blue
Eyes" by A. P. Carter, copyright © 1929, copyright renewed 1957 by Peer
International Corporation. All rights reserved. International copyright secured.
Reprinted by permission of Peer International Corporation.

Stage Three Songs: Excerpt from "Heard It on the X" by Billy F. Gibbons, Dusty
Hill, and Frank Beard, copyright © Stage Three Songs (ASCAP). All rights reserved.
Reprinted by permission of Stage Three Songs.

Library of Congress Cataloging-in-Publication Data

Brock, Pope.
Charlatan: America's most dangerous huckster, the man who
pursued him, and the age of flimflam / Pope Brock.
p. cm.
1. Brinkley, John R., 1885–1942. 2. Quacks and quackery—
United States—History. I. Title.
R730.B76 2008
615.8'56—dc22   2007010074

ISBN 978-0-307-33989-8

Printed in the United States of America

DESIGN BY LEONARD W. HENDERSON

10 9 8 7 6 5 4 3 2

First Paperback Edition

For my daughters,
Molly and Hannah

Truth, sir, is a cow that will yield such people no more milk,
and so they are gone to milk the bull.

— SAMUEL JOHNSON

Charlatan

Prologue

E very member of the panel showed up for the demonstration, but the carload traveling from Kansas City was delayed by bad roads. It was nearly eleven A.M. before the stragglers finally arrived in Milford, a sketchy little town with an extraordinarily large post office on the banks of the Republican River.

Nearing the clinic, the driver looked for some shade to park in. There wasn't any. That summer had been the hottest ever recorded in Kansas, and instead of the usual jungles of corn, there were miles of shriveled stalks and cracked earth stretching off in all directions, nothing growing to speak of but a few cane-thin cottonwood trees. The birdcage shadow of the radio tower looked painted on the ground.

The screen door banged, and a couple of staffers came outside to welcome them. In a conference room the late arrivals found their fellow delegates and, even better, the lemonade.

Shortly afterward Dr. J. F. Hassig, president of the Kansas State Medical Board, and more than twenty colleagues and reporters clattered up the narrow-walled stairs to the second floor. Leading the way was the clinic's second-in-command, Horatius Dwight Osborn, a symbol to some of doglike devotion, since Osborn had only one ear— or to be more precise, only one ear left.

The herd moved along the corridor. As they peered into patients' rooms, looks of reserved surprise were discernible among the doctors. Envy perhaps? (A reporter noted that the facilities here "surpassed for modernity, convenience and luxury the places in which their own carving was done.") There were sixteen private rooms, no two the same, but each graced with an overstuffed davenport, heartening artwork, bits of bric-a-brac: Mrs. Brinkley's touch, no doubt. Country music floated from bedside radios. What the visitors were seeing, in short, was a rare marriage of charm and the healing arts, and to have such a renowned physician—for Dr. John R. Brinkley, M.D., Ph.D., M.C., LL.D., D.P.H., Sc.D., was now a world figure—choose such an unassuming little town as Milford, Kansas, for his medical mecca made its personal feel all the more personal.

Inspection complete, the group returned to the first floor. There they mused among the exhibits in the so-called trophy room, where the doctor kept some of his odder removals on display.

Then through a window someone spied their host—the Burbank of Humanity, the Chinese called him—heading toward the building. Brisk, rather short, with a sandy Vandyke, Dr. Brinkley was dressed in full medical regalia and a surgeon's cap. He carried his mask in his hand. In the downstairs hall he shook hands with several of his guests. He seemed quite calm: a vessel of intellect oblivious to pressure. Of course he had performed his famous procedure hundreds of times but rarely with such a distinguished audience.

Another handclasp, a wave of thanks to the rest, and the doctor disappeared into the operating room. An aide passed out sterile robes to everyone. When the last bow was tied, another assistant pushed back the door.

"This way, gentlemen."

It was a tight fit. The twelve members of the state medical board, four other observing surgeons, and of course the press with their marginal manners all had to wedge themselves into the room as best they could, taking care to leave sufficient space for Brinkley's staff—and for the man on the table, whom the doctor now introduced.

"This is Mr. X," he said.

There were mumbled hellos. Mr. X—identified as a fifty-five-year-old mail carrier—smiled but did not speak.

At a nod from her husband Mrs. Brinkley, wearing spectacles and a trapezoidal cap, came forward and gave the patient a local anesthetic, injecting him twice just below the waistline. Other aides toyed with the umbrella-frame lighting system overhead, tilting and focusing each bulb till the doctor was satisfied.

Then an orderly brought up the goat from the basement.

Why the goat was being kept downstairs was never explained. Ordinarily they resided in pens outside in the fresh air—even now the baaing of others could be heard through the open window. No matter; what counted was that this particular goat, a three- to four-week-old male, was Mr. X's personal choice.

The trembling animal was placed, hoofs clattering, on a side table. Then Mrs. Brinkley drew a chair up close to it and sat. Her fingertips, freshly dipped in antiseptic, played in a tray of shining instruments. A nurse stood by with a nest of gauze.

While the orderly held the goat's head, the doctor's wife brushed part of its underbelly with Mercurochrome. Then she picked up a small pair of scissors.

Someone down the hall heard "the bleating of the goat ringing through the corridors."

The nurse held out her hands, and Mrs. Brinkley deposited the testicles one by one onto the gauze. As the doctor donned rubber gloves, the glands were transferred to a stainless-steel tray and placed beside him.

The patient lay lightly strapped down, a wet towel on his forehead. Dr. Brinkley inspected each gland closely, then raised his mask and set to work.

"No one who was at the institution for this unusual display of a surgical performance went away doubting that [Brinkley] has nerve," reported the *Kansas City Journal-Post*.

Aside from Brinkley himself, those closest to the table were Drs. Nesselrode, Edgerton, Orr, and Carr, the four "official spectators" charged with making a scientific report on what they saw. Dr. Brinkley, however, took care that everyone had a clear view, standing back from time to time to explain another step of the so-called four-phase compound operation. Dr. Hassig, who also took precise notes, saw the doctor first make twin incisions in the patient's scrotum, "slitting it and injecting each way through a blunt needle about two cc's of one-half percent Mercurochrome," after which a fresh goat testis was implanted on each side and then sutured to the "loose tissue."

The procedure was supposed to take ten minutes. At fifteen, the spectators began to exchange glances. Dr. Brinkley abandoned explanations and bent more closely to his work. Twenty minutes, thirty. Although he betrayed no alarm, more than one of those watching felt that first touch of dread at the temples, a faraway fear that the patient might . . . Should someone intervene? Doubtless sensing the uneasiness, the doctor paused briefly to lower his mask and give a smile of reassurance. Then he returned to his labors.

A full forty-five minutes passed before he drew the last catgut stitch and stepped back. Assisted by a nurse, Mr. X sat up dizzily, swung his legs over the side, pitched a bit to the right, but was caught and steadied. He took a few breaths. Then he slid off the table and, with a drunkard's dignity, exited the room.

Dr. Brinkley took off his mask. While pronouncing the operation a success, he spoke candidly about the unexpected complications. He suggested without quite saying so that they had been a lucky thing, allowing him to demonstrate skills and resourcefulness that might otherwise have gone untested. "If any of you gentlemen have patients that you feel need attention of this kind," he concluded suavely, "we will be glad to handle them here."

The members of the Kansas State Medical Board thanked him and took their leave, repairing en masse to the Barfell House in nearby Junction City for lunch.

Forty-eight hours later they unanimously revoked his license to practice on grounds of "gross immorality and unprofessional conduct." The Kansas Supreme Court, which rejected his appeal, saluted him thus: "Being an empiric without moral sense, and having acted according to the ethical standards of an imposter, the licensee has perfected an organized charlatanism . . . quite beyond the invention of the humble mountebank."

The *Kansas City Star* pronounced the eulogy: "The superquack of Milford is finished."

Their confidence was drastically misplaced.

1

In the period before the First World War, the Reinhardt brothers, Willis and Wallace, owned a thriving chain of anatomical museums: the London Medical Institute, the Paris Medical Institute, the Heidelberg, the Copenhagen, and so forth. Located in Des Moines, Fort Wayne, East St. Louis, and other towns throughout the Midwest, they were devoted to the documentation and cure of "men's secret diseases." Most had big display windows facing the street, and what the Reinhardts put in those windows was the talk of the industry. Their most celebrated exhibit, in Minneapolis, was entitled "The Dying Custer."

He lay like Saint Sebastian, bristling with arrows, in a lavish three-dimensional tableau. Redskins, corpses, and plaster vultures added richness to the scene, but what kept passersby bunched at the window, staring in for minutes on end, was the slow, rhythmic heaving of Custer's chest. They gazed till their own breathing fell into sync—it was irresistible—and that gave the Reinhardts' message time to go to work. True, Custer's connection to impotence may have been largely metaphorical, but to a certain fretful portion of the populace it struck home. Power gone, youth destroyed—but not yet, not quite yet. Inside this building there was even hope for Yellow Hair.

Mixing terror and hope was the Reinhardts' stock-in-trade. Their window in Gary, Indiana—again designed by their visionary house artist, Monsieur Brouillard—featured a diorama of a doctor and nurse trying to save a syphilitic baby with the help of a wheezing resuscitator. But displays alone, no matter how artful, didn't make the

Reinhardt twins tops in their field. From their headquarters at the Vienna Medical Institute in Chicago, where they rode herd on some three dozen franchises, they enforced levels of standardization and quality control remarkably ahead of their time. Starting with their training of salesmen: nobody worked for the Reinhardts without first graduating from the "instantaneous medical college" at the home office. This was followed by more training at the Gary branch, where each recruit was given a white coat, asked to grow a Vandyke, and made to practice his patter as if it were Gilbert and Sullivan. Only then were real customers released upon them. Serving as exhibition guides, the floor men were expected to nail 20 percent of all prospects—eight out of an average forty walk-ins a day—or look for another job. The manager of each institute sent headquarters a daily financial report in triplicate.

Admission was free at all these places. The abba-dabba juice was not. Bottles of it were on sale at the exit, a fabled elixir guaranteed to soothe, stimulate, inflate, reinstate, backdate, laminate, and in general make "the withered bough quicken and grow green again," while at the same time curing and/or preventing the clap; it adapted to the needs of the customer. What was in it? What was in any of them? What was in Dr. Raphael's Cordial Invigorant, America's first big virility tonic in the 1850s, whose royal Arabian formula was made vastly more potent by the "magical influence of modern Astrologers"? What was the recipe for Baume de Vie, Elixir Renovans, the Syrop Vitae of Anthony Bellou, the Glorious Spagyric of Jone Case, or any of the others in lands and ages stretching back to the dawn of time? For the record, the Reinhardts' tonic contained three ingredients— alcohol, sugar, and a dash of "Aqua Missourianas quantitat sufficiat ad cong II"—but this is pedantry.

Big as they were, the Reinhardts still had plenty of competition. Independents with similar rackets were out there grubbing in the twilight, men like Dr. Burke of Knoxville, Tennessee, who in 1907 was running his own small shop with the help of an assistant, Dr. John Brinkley.

Young Brinkley was a likely lad of twenty-two. To call him a doctor was, in the strictest sense, inaccurate, but if the white coat reassured people, the healing had begun. In truth he was the floor man and he worked on commission. Brinkley would study a prospect as he came through the door, then materialize—not too soon—at his elbow. The young physician chatted, he chuckled, he took a grave interest; he showed the man around. Soon the two were passing along the main line of exhibits: a stage-by-stage depiction of the male member in syphilitic decline. It spoke for itself. With each new cabinet the organ grew more deformed and the colors changed. Perhaps leprosy was mentioned by way of comparison.

In the last room the customer met The Boy.

It was known by that name throughout the trade, and every "free educational anatomical institute" worth its salt had one. The scene was replayed countless times: while the salesman hung back, or bent to tie his shoe, the customer approached a rectangular pillar walled in glass. It was pitch-dark inside. The mark moved toward it cautiously, perhaps glancing back at his guide for the go-ahead, peered in close trying to see what was in there—and then the lights blazed on full, and the grinning wax face of an idiot sprang into view. Horrifying as it was, the warning above it was even worse:

LOST MANHOOD

The customer knew then that he wasn't just looking at a vile mask with dripping yellow eyes. He was looking at the future. He was looking at himself.

After this bit of venereal kabuki—"the convincer," in quack talk—the rest was usually easy. As Dr. Burke sat at a desk, possibly lost in a medical tome, Dr. Brinkley brought the poor sinner forward and introduced him. Burke gave him an "instant consultation" ("Are you ever thirsty?" "Do you sometimes suffer from fatigue?"—warning signs all) and produced a bottle of peerless tonic, which the man was assured would save his organ and probably his life. The price was almost as big a shock as The Boy, between ten and twenty dollars, but who in his right mind would economize at a time like this? Moments later the customer was standing in the alley with the hooey in his hand and the door shut firmly behind him.

How much satisfaction Brinkley felt at such moments is unknown. The greatest quacks never gloat for long; when deception is the drug, there's no building up a supply. Besides, he had so much ambition that working in two tatty rooms with a substandard Boy could have been depressing at times.

On the other hand, he might have taken pride in having gotten so far so young. Brinkley came from the tiny town of Beta, North Carolina, tucked in the Great Smokies not far from the Tennessee line. Like his neighbors, he grew up on a hilly little farm that produced mostly rocks. He ate mush and greens and lashed gunnysacks to his feet for winter boots. The thick forests and hard climbs, the rainy days when bowls of fog gathered in the valleys, the strangers scarce as hen's teeth: all this conspired to make the outside world seem little more than a rumor, so it was natural that most people, if they started out there, stayed put.

Not Brinkley. "Kind of a recklesslike boy," one neighbor called him. "Lively as a cricket," another said. And all the while he burned with a bitter fire, and he dreamed. ("I thought of John Brinkley freeing the slaves," he said later, "John Brinkley illuminating the world, John Brinkley facing an assassin's bullet for the sake of his people, John Brinkley healing the sick.") But with the slaves freed, the world lit, and nobody caring enough about him to kill him, he chose number four—sort of. First he married Sally Wike, a spitfire from a neighboring farm, as eager as he was to escape the prison of the mountains. Then "he got up a little play," as Mrs. Ann Bennett, who boarded them briefly, recalled it, "and he and his wife and some more people went on the road from town to town, you know, giving little plays."

He sang and he danced and he healed. Barely twenty, Brinkley got his precocious start touring as a type of medicine man known as a Quaker doctor. Though, in the general run of Quakers, specialty numbers were almost unknown, some itinerant quacks in those days liked to impersonate them, trading on their legendary rectitude. Some folks saw through the act, but it hardly mattered. Fooling some of the people all of the time and all of the people some of the time was plenty.

They usually performed at night. A platform was unfolded and torches placed at each corner as the audience gathered, drawn by handbills and word of mouth. While there is no specific record of a Brinkley performance, there was a set pattern to most Quaker-doctor shows. First a fiddler or a dancer got the crowd warmed up. A short morality play followed, in which a noble head of house or ringleted female died pathetically for lack of a miracle tonic, identified by name. Finally the physician himself (Brinkley) shot onstage in a dinner-plate hat, cutaway coat, and pious pants that buttoned up the sides, theeing and thouing, singing and selling, waving a bottle of Ayer's Cathartic Pills. Or maybe Burdock Blood Bitters or Aunt Fanny's Worm Candy. One thing was for sure, whatever it was cured whatever you had.

With his unerring nose for where the money was, Brinkley had already become an American archetype: the quack on the boards. For in our nation with its special genius for swindle—where swampland, beefsteak mines, and tickets to nonexistent attractions practically sell themselves—medical fraud had always been the king of cons. At the 1893 World's Fair in Chicago, a man dressed as a cowboy appeared onstage and strangled rattlesnakes by the dozen. He called what came out of them snake oil. People bought it.

Of course quacks have flourished in all ages and cultures, for nothing shows reason the door like cures for things. Unlike most scams, which target greed, quackery fires deeper into Jungian universals: our fear of death, our craving for miracles. When we see night approaching, nearly all of us are rubes.

Still, there has probably never been a more quack-prone and quack-infested country than the United States. Flocking west with the pioneers, they struck in one town, vanished to the next, and taught their tricks to others. Dupes were as common as passenger pigeons. Many Americans viewed hospitals, sometimes with justice, as tricked-up funeral homes and doctors as crooks who had a financial stake in keeping them sick.

But quacks weren't just accepted; they were joyously embraced, thanks to a perverse seam in the American mind stretching back almost to the dawn of the republic.

It first appeared in the early nineteenth century. In the heady days of Jacksonian democracy, that delirious celebration of the ordinary, the nation's elite—preachers, doctors, lawyers—were overthrown (at least mentally) with an abandon reminiscent of the French Revolution. Suddenly, to be educated was to be despised. Now, when it came to physicians, Americans not only tolerated but demanded incompetence. So high was the common man exalted that state governments, all but three, actually repealed licensing requirements for doctors. In midcentury educator Lemuel Shattuck, asked by the Massachusetts legislature to conduct a sanitary survey of that state, reported back: "Any one, male or female, learned or ignorant, an honest man or a knave, can assume the name of physician, and 'practice' upon any one, to cure or to kill, as either may happen, without accountability. It's a free country!"

The result of all this deregulation was the quack equivalent of the Oklahoma Land Rush, with effects that lasted for generations to come. Legitimate doctors had difficulty fighting back, their own record being spotty at best. Take Dr. Benjamin Rush, friend to the founders, signer of the Declaration of Independence, and by common consent the father of American medicine, who for many years after his death remained the nation's best-known physician. Hardworking, honest, a man who took his role as medical counselor to the nation seriously, he was also a virtual death machine, as grossly misguided as he was sincere. Rush favored bombing the body with mercury-laced calomel (which caused rampant diarrhea, bleeding of the gums, and uncontrolled drooling), blistering with hot irons (pain to no purpose), tobacco-smoke enemas, and bleeding by the pint. Some remember

him today as the man who murdered George Washington, albeit unintentionally. Of course every evil has its upside: thanks in part to men
like Rush, degenerative diseases of the heart, liver, kidneys, and so
forth were almost unknown because so few people lived long enough
to contract them.

So just who were the quacks? In this melee of plagues and poisons
did it even matter? Granted, the people who bought pills against
earthquakes were probably wasting their money, but when a man like
Elisha Perkins (a contemporary of Dr. Rush) came along with his
"galvanic tractors," fussing over the body with some hocus-pocus
and two metal rods, at least he held with Hippocrates and did no
harm. Like Dr. Rush, Dr. Perkins believed in what he was doing. Both
were wrong, yet the one was honored and the other condemned.
Given history like this, it becomes easier to understand why the
people John Brinkley played to—especially the sick and frightened—
were willing to give that youngster onstage the benefit of the doubt.

Confederates passed through the crowd laden with bottles of
medicine for sale, while he cried up its vitalizing force, efficacious
effluvium, and low, low price.

"All sold out, Doctor!"

"Bless you, my friends!"

The little troupe disbanded within a few months, and Brinkley
never sang or danced for the rest of his career. Though he learned
some important lessons, which he would later apply on the world
stage, he was a faux scientist of the twentieth century, not a clown of
the nineteenth. Working for Dr. Burke, his next step, at least put him
in the right coat. But like his early role model, Abraham Lincoln, his
ambition was a little engine that knew no rest, and in 1908 Brinkley
moved on again, heading north this time toward the big city.

2

One thing at least would have been familiar: the fog that dragged, Smoky Mountain–style, across the grain elevators along the Chicago River. Some days it swallowed up portions of the city. It settled in doorways and ballooned slowly from passageways and alleys, mixing with steam and coal smoke, through which pedestrians burst as if out of a dream.

The city threw light at the problem. Along with snake oil, its recent world's fair had showcased Edison's great breakthrough, and ever since then Chicago had been his best customer. It became a city, one resident said, of "incredibly long lanes of street-lamps, up and down the slopes; light everywhere; light lavished and wasted; as much candle-power used in a week as the whole nation once used in a year." And it was by this light, on an evening's prowl along the Gold Coast, that Brinkley first beheld the world he had always dreamed of.

Fronting the already poisoned waters of Lake Michigan stood a receiving line of mansions: Rhine castles, gothic fortresses, medieval watchtowers, interrupted by hedges and open stables and the rumps of the best horses. Not everything was in the best of taste, but that was the point. The wealth of this new aristocracy—the lords of buttons and dry goods, the kings of pork—was gaudy and unembarrassed. You could smell it on the breeze. The Libbeys, the Swifts, and the Armours had alchemized seventy-five miles of sliding stockyard sewage into a sort of best-guess version of high society: theme parties and soirees, top hats and hourglass gowns, French toques with egret feathers and dog collars of pearls. To Brinkley this was the definition of money well spent.

He liked other things about Chicago. The same perch near the top of the Mississippi that made the city a hub for livestock (and later liquor and the blues) also made it a natural gathering ground for quacks. In Brinkley's line alone, the virility racket, opportunities abounded. Along with the Reinhardt twins, the Packers Product Company was based here, manufacturers of Orchis Extract, the alleged essence of rams' testicles. The company letterhead carried a picture of the Union Stock Yards at the top, with Armour headquarters visible. Packers had no affiliation with Armour; the purpose was simply to link the concepts of Orchis and big meat. At the rival Animal Therapy Company, when its two partners quarreled over profits, one walked across the hall and put a bullet between the eyes of the other—quackery, Chicago-style.

But Brinkley wasn't interested in all this, at least for now. He had come to town with another purpose: to go to medical school. It's conceivable he intended, however briefly, to go straight. More likely he understood that the success he dreamed of required the sheen of respectability and a bigger toolbox. Either way he had to work quickly. Married to Sally, with two daughters and a third child on the way, he had responsibilities.

What kind of school should he attend?

For many in his position the answer was obvious. The American Medical Association, the physicians' mother church of respectability, was headquartered in Chicago, and several mainstream schools operated there under its protection and scrutiny. These institutions drew legions of foursquare, impeccably conservative students—men like Morris Fishbein, who arrived in town not long after Brinkley. A roly-poly youth from Indianapolis, Fishbein was the son of a glassware merchant who had emigrated from eastern Europe. Morris had been inspired to become a doctor, at least in part, by something he had seen regularly in the park near his home: people sitting on benches after visits to Dr. Benjamin Bye, a neighborhood cancer quack. Bye specialized in cancers of the face and neck, which he treated with a caustic paste. Fishbein never forgot, as he later wrote, "the disastrous appearance of those patients"—the heads bandaged, the blood soaking through. Now he was about to enter Rush Medical College, which (though named for a man disastrous in his own right) was the city's oldest medical school, one of the best respected, with close ties to the University of Chicago and blessed by the AMA.

Brinkley, on the other hand, had applied nowhere ahead of time. With his instinct for coloring outside the lines, he was more inclined to browse. He had a number of options.

The AMA-approved schools, like Rush Medical College, taught a type of medicine called allopathy. Dominant throughout the country, this approach was founded on scientific experiment—that is, drugs developed in the lab—and surgery. But the allopathics were hardly in charge. Other accredited and successful schools as splintered as the sects of Christianity variously preached the gospels of osteopathy, chiropractic, homeopathy, herbs, and more. The AMA loathed and denounced them all, but in this it was like the angry upstairs neighbor who keeps coming down to complain about the noise. Nobody listened. Since the founding of the American Medical Association in 1847—a reaction to the free-for-all of nonlicensing— the process of becoming a doctor had changed mightily, but the present system simply swapped one form of chaos for another. Now in most states each branch of medicine had its own licensing board. It would have been hard to purposely design a system more lax and corrupt.

Brinkley shopped around and selected Bennett Eclectic Medical College. With about five thousand practitioners around the country, 4 percent of licensed physicians, eclectic medicine relied chiefly on herbal remedies. Not everything about it was quackish. Eclecticism had always opposed treatments like bleeding and mercury even when more respectable disciplines had not, and some of its theories on plant use were ahead of their time. But it also tolerated a lot of woolly-headed guesswork—"old grandmother and witch-doctor" treatments, the AMA called them—which made its academic coursework easier and cheaper than most.

Brinkley borrowed the twenty-five-dollar entry fee from a loan shark and started classes on June 26, 1908.

Student by day, telegraph operator by night, he grabbed ten-cent dinners at nightfall downtown at Pittsburgh Joe's. It was a punishing routine, but no one ever said he was lazy. He drank, and as time went on he drank more, like a lot of other people in Chicago. The city's livestock-flavored water, courtesy of the stockyards, sickened or killed a disproportionate number of citizens and drove others into a sort of defensive alcoholism. At least it was a popular excuse.

For three years he kept it all going, but the work and the liquor wore him down, and he grew increasingly morose. There he sat nuzzling steins in the company of vagrants and pickled eggs while the swells were sipping Benedictine and gazing out the window at their sailboats. Meanwhile his wife, Sally, was developing into a harpy of Greek proportions. The problem wasn't so much growing differences between them as it was discovering they simply didn't like each other. Sally had his number, though. She could see by his brooding that he was gearing up for some big change; he had a trick, she later said, of "always pitying himself to gain confidence." When he quit school with a year still to go, Brinkley said it was because he didn't have the money, but he might have done the same anyway. To a certain kind of mind, graduation is cheating.

Two years later, on an early spring evening in 1913, he stood in the fabled bar of the Brevoort Hotel.

He was in downtown Chicago, no more than half a mile from where his odyssey had begun, but in the time between he had rambled all over the Midwest. After shedding his wife and children—he and Sally didn't even bother to divorce—he had hit the road. What he was looking for, he didn't know. For two years he dodged bill collectors and rode the rails and drank when he could afford it. He spent months lurking in St. Louis doing nothing in particular. Finally in February 1913, at age twenty-seven, he returned to Chicago with an itch for fame but still no plan.

Things had changed since he'd been away. Chicago was in the grips of an antivice crusade targeting the barrelhouse joints and all-night oyster bars. But he was done with all that anyway. From here on, if he had to lurk, he would lurk at the top.

The Brevoort was one of the finest hotels in the city. Its lobby was like the Harvard Club swollen to fifty times normal size, with maroon leather armchairs and epic chandeliers. Adjoining it was the bar, a masculine preserve ornate even for the period. Done in cream, rose, green, and gold, with mirrored rectangular columns, it outrococoed most of old Europe. The bar itself, set in the center, was round and embedded with crystal snowflakes.

Financially it was way over Brinkley's head, but spiritually it was perfect. Here gathered the men he most admired, the rough and rowdy capitalists with their matching paunches and dollar cigars. The drinks were stiff and the talk was the roar of prosperity.

It's not surprising that Brinkley and James Crawford should have found each other here. They were two sore thumbs, two aspirers dressed not quite well enough for the room. Each was alone. Possibly Crawford's having only one arm spoke to the physician in Brinkley, or maybe they recognized the grifter in each other's eyes.

They had a drink together. Crawford was twenty-three years old, from Oxford, Mississippi. He said he'd been the victim of a hunting accident—though even with two arms he hadn't been any world-beater, as Brinkley soon figured out.

Still, he was company. Even better, he could be of use.

3

When Brinkley and Crawford teamed up, quackery was in crisis. The first shock had come in October 1905 when *Collier's* introduced a pioneering series of articles by Samuel Hopkins Adams. Titled "The Great American Fraud," it began by promising a "full explanation and exposure of patent medicine methods and the harm done to the public by this industry." Then, to the consternation of the country, Adams delivered.

"Gullible America," he wrote, "will spend this year some seventy-five million dollars in the purchase of patent medicines. In consideration of this sum it will swallow huge quantities of alcohol, an appalling amount of opiates and narcotics, a wide assortment of varied drugs ranging from powerful and dangerous heart depressants to insidious liver stimulants; and, far in excess of other ingredients, undiluted fraud."

Over the course of eleven articles he flayed the patent-medicine business, all the way back to Benjamin Franklin's mother-in-law and her "well-known Ointment for the ITCH." Primarily, though, he named names in the present: 264 culpable companies and individuals. As curatives most of what they sold was worthless at best (ketchup started life as a patent medicine), but Adams saved his greatest venom for those whose reckless dispensing of cocaine and opium "stupefies helpless babies and makes criminals of our young men and harlots of our young women." He also disclosed the alcohol content of famous brands like Paine's Celery Compound (21 percent) and Hostetter's Stomach Bitters (44.3 percent). The bestselling of the bunch was Peruna, "the most prominent proprietary nostrum in the country," manufactured by a Dr. S. B. Hartman of Cincinnati. Favored by bridge-playing old ladies and other discreet alcoholics, it had spawned the term *Peruna drunk* and been banned from reservations by the Bureau of Indian Affairs, while producing imitators like Pe-ru-vi-na, P-Ru-Na, Perina, and Anurep. Within a year of Adams's exposé, Hartman was told by the IRS either to put real medicine in his product or "open a bar."

But the most important response to the *Collier's* series (together with *The Jungle,* Upton Sinclair's exposé of the Chicago stockyards) was the passing of the first Pure Food and Drug Act in 1906. The law was characteristically congressional; that is, it left rat holes for industry to hide in. Nevertheless, as Lady Bracknell observed, "ignorance is like a delicate, exotic fruit; touch it, and the bloom is gone." Now that the public had been alerted to the scourge of patent medicines, the golden age for manufacturers was over. Right in step with *Collier's,* the AMA hired a former high-school science teacher from Milwaukee, Arthur J. Cramp, to head a new antifraud unit of its own.

What this meant for Brinkley and Crawford, as they plotted the future, was that the old tonic wheeze would no longer suffice. They needed something with more snap, more pizzazz, something worthy of the age of Edison.

Time: a summer day in 1913. Place: Greenville, South Carolina. Amid the clutter of signs along Main Street, the newest is a discreet bronze doorplate at the bottom of a flight of stairs:

GREENVILLE ELECTRO MEDIC DOCTORS

The office is over a shoe store near the corner of Coffee and Main. Farther along, a brick emporium sells lace, ribbons, mule shoes, and molasses, and out back of the restaurant these sweltering afternoons, a couple of the willfully unemployed are usually chewing tobacco and taking long squirts at the bees that hover over the trash. Aside from Shoeless Joe Jackson, the local boy made good, Greenville isn't known for much of anything except maybe its mud—a red, shoe-sucking muck that some people on wet days swear is carnivorous.

The partners had traveled first to Knoxville, Tennessee, where Brinkley's old boss and mentor still ran his syphilis museum. For two weeks Dr. Burke graciously taught Crawford the finer points of quack bookkeeping and customer psychology, in return for which, once he was back on the road, Crawford started calling himself Dr. Burke for credit purposes. Brinkley became Blakely. They had taken soundings in several towns before settling on this one.

First stop was the barbershop for shaves and haircuts. Then, smelling prosperously of bay rum, they went all over Greenville establishing credit accounts. Clothes, furniture, office space, and phones were bought, rented, or arranged for; the two also charmed drugs and medical supplies out of the pharmacist across the street, an elderly party who dispensed mercury pills for depression and still bled the occasional customer with leeches off the back shelf. Next to him these fellows from up north looked like tomorrow's headlines. Besides, even in defiantly backward Greenville—where some folks still insisted that if God had wanted that bridge over the Reedy River, he would have put it there himself—the fad for healing with electricity had been gaining ground. Electric ointments were selling across the country, electric hairbrushes, electric corsets, electric belts; there were even ads for electric food. (People either didn't notice or didn't care that Thomas A. Edison Jr., creator of the Magno-Electric Vitalizer, had been arrested for fraud in 1904.) Now, thanks to Brinkley and Crawford, Greenville had its very own electric doctors. Their ads in the *Daily News* were a frank challenge to every man to look inside himself, or just look down:

Are You a Manly Man Full of Vigor?

The answer in many cases was happily no. Each morning brought another bunch of doleful shufflers into the office of Drs. Blakely and Burke. From bankers to farmers, from young bucks to the old and dim, all crov

mute, under

walked acros

whose Southe

who had also

Dr. Burke

his palm for tw

passed on into t

ing injecting col

was electric mec

The pair ski

altogether is unl

forty merchants v

Crawford said

Mississippi, the pa

enough considerin

law enforcement was difficult and rare; it u

der to even put it in motion. But by bei

Brinkley and Crawford had infuria

zens who, as the *Daily News* pu

thetic which the Electric Me

worse than losing the m

Sheriff Hendrix

all over the cou

up with pho

Brinkley

which

...and steamboats on the perimeter and a downtown teeming with straw boaters, striped ties, and so many women in long white dresses it looked like a city full of brides.

The perfect place for Brinkley to meet Minerva Telitha Jones. Perhaps a former acquaintance of Crawford's, Minnie was twenty-one, the daughter of a prominent local physician, and she liked to go dancing on some of those riverboats. She had the odd knack, evident in photographs, of looking glamorous one moment, gap-toothed hillbilly the next, and good either way. At least Brinkley thought so.

On August 23, 1913, just four days after they met, they were married at the old Peabody Hotel. Dr. and Mrs. Tiberius Gracchus Jones and Minnie's brother, also Tiberius, attended. Crawford was best man. Brinkley didn't spoil the happy day by telling anyone, including Minnie, that he already had a wife.

He did tell her during their honeymoon out west. Minnie was willing to work the problem out together, but when she informed her father on their return, he was fit to be tied.

Then the Greenville sheriff appeared.

Statistically this was little short of amazing. Interstate pursuit by

...sually took at least a mur-
...ing so good at what they did,
...ted the dozens of Greenville citi-
...it, "fell victims to the hot air anaes-
...dics administered." The humiliation was
...oney, and the marks wanted revenge.

...Rector mailed wanted posters to police stations
...try offering a forty-dollar reward, and he followed
...e calls. Finally the authorities in Knoxville recognized
...apparently through his connection to the real Dr. Burke,
...led to a concentrated search in Tennessee.

On December 8, 1913, Sheriff Rector clapped handcuffs on the new groom—who blamed everything on Crawford—and took him back to Greenville on the train. They journeyed overnight, shackled together. In the shadows other passengers snored, ate out of shoeboxes, or bought fried chicken and ginger cakes through the windows at station stops. No offer was made to feed the prisoner.

The Greenville jail, better known as Little Siberia, was a stone pile next to a weedy vacant lot strewn with empty bottles. One of the grimy little windows facing the street was broken, and a pillow had been stuffed in it to keep out the cold. The cells were on the second floor, and here the weather poured in; no panes, only iron bars.

The ex-fugitive was charged with forgery and practicing medicine without a license.

If huddling on an iron cot over Christmas far from his bride was gall and wormwood to Brinkley, at least he didn't suffer alone. Thanks to information he supplied, Crawford was tracked down in Kansas City where he was working as a bread salesman. Ten days after Brinkley's arrival, Crawford was brought in and put in a cell across the hall. Each was held on three thousand dollars bond.

Married just four months to the girl of his dreams, then exposed as a bigamist, forger, and quack. Perhaps he had a Scarlett O'Hara moment. From here on out he would prove wonderfully adept at staying out of jail.

4

In 1912 Morris Fishbein graduated from Rush Medical College. He had thrived in school as a favorite of important senior faculty like Dr. Max Thorek, a Hungarian who was chief of surgery at a top Chicago hospital. Now the young man was ready for . . . what? He couldn't decide. Hesitating between pathology and pediatrics, he spent a few months on staff at the McCormick Institute for Infectious Diseases without choosing a specialty. But as it turned out, he didn't need to; he was about to leave patient care forever. In August 1913 (the month Brinkley was married) Fishbein was offered a temporary position as assistant to the editor of the *Journal of the American Medical Association,* largely on the strength of his shorthand. This job, which he took as a stopgap, would propel him into his long and improbable career as the great quack buster of his day, and later the hellhound on Brinkley's trail.

At *JAMA*'s modest offices on Dearborn Street, the twenty-four-year-old Fishbein brought his gobbling intelligence and photographic memory to the great medical questions of the day. He talked fast and he talked a lot ("because I have so much to say"). If he was told some topic in the magazine might bore the public, "his eyes bulge[d] unbelievingly," a colleague said. Already balding and potato shaped, Fishbein struck a visitor as "precocity personified. . . . He was not yet, when I met him, Mr. A.M.A., but he gave the impression that it wouldn't be long before he would be."

Fishbein himself was impressed by Arthur Cramp, the man hired in the wake of the *Collier's* series to head up the AMA's Bureau of

Investigation. Soft-spoken, fastidious, a bird-watcher in his off-hours, Cramp struck some as a bit of a milquetoast. But in Milwaukee, where he'd taught school, his young daughter had died at the hands of a quack, and ever since then he had devoted his life to destroying the whole fraternity. Since 1906 exposés of medical charlatans had poured from his pen. Still he had an engaging sense of the absurd: before savaging each new target, he liked to read a chapter of *Alice in Wonderland*. He said it put him in the right mood.

One day Cramp showed the new assistant editor his enormous patent medicine collection. It was like walking into a cave of skulls or Jefferson's wine cellar: even Fishbein fell silent. On Cramp's desk stood a bottle of his current quarry, Wine of Cardui, a 38-proof "uterine sedative" which claimed to "raise the fallen womb." The two men wound up collaborating on the *JAMA* article that exposed it as a fraud, the start of a partnership that would last for more than twenty years. Starting out as mentor, Cramp eventually came to play Billy Strayhorn to Fishbein's Ellington, the offstage alter ego feeding and boosting the performance of the maestro.

The sheer number of bad checks actually worked in the electromedics' favor. Lawyers consolidated the complaints into a single settlement proposal (several thousand dollars), and the Greenville merchants accepted it. Crawford supplied most of the money to spring them, his partner little or nothing. Minnie's father contributed two hundred dollars by wire. Either his daughter's pleas had touched him, or he had the gift of prescience: later on when Brinkley achieved his huge success, he put the old man and Minnie's brother and sister all on the payroll. There is no record of Greenville's swindled patients getting anything, probably because they were too shy to speak up.

The deal was signed on December 31. "In their hurry to get out of the city," the *Daily News* reported, "Brinkley and Crawford left their luggage at the jail." The partnership was finished.

In Memphis, Minnie was waiting, as faithful as Juliet and tough as nails. For the next three years the still-not-quite-legal couple roamed through Kansas and Arkansas, while Brinkley scratched a living as a traveling medico. Eventually, like the scarecrow in *The Wizard of Oz,* he had everything but a diploma, so he bought one. On May 7, 1915, the Eclectic Medical University of Kansas City presented him with a certificate signed by its president, Dr. Date R. Alexander. To become an alumnus of E.M.U. (later described in court proceedings as "vague, obliging and long defunct") cost Brinkley one hundred dollars and got him licensed in eight states.

First he tried setting up as a GP in Judsonia, Arkansas. He had a little trick there for trying to drum up business, renting a horse now and then at the livery stable and galloping out of town as if on an urgent call, but it didn't work and they had to move on. His divorce came through at last, however, and he and Minnie officially remarried, formalizing what the years would prove: how much they loved each other.

For a few weeks in 1916 Brinkley served as "physician and clerk" at a Kansas City meatpacking plant. In idle hours he watched billy goats copulate in their pens, just minutes away from slaughter: sure food for the philosopher. He was struck, as he later said, by their "considerable lubricity." A meat inspector told him that compared with other livestock goats got sick the least.

As he gazed at them, Brinkley was tortured by formless ambition. He was thirty-one years old now. Would he ever tear his way out of this moonless obscurity? How he longed to become a giant like the great Dr. Abrams—Albert Abrams of San Francisco—the gold standard then, the colossus of quackery. Sporting a classic Vandyke and pince-nez with black ribbon, Abrams had first gained fame with his book *Spondylotherapy* in 1910, wherein he revealed that disease could be diagnosed and cured by "a steady, rapid percussing or hammering of the spine." Soon he added a new wrinkle, the "rheostatic dynamizer," a box with wires in it. First a drop of the patient's blood was placed inside. Then more wires were run to the head of someone else, a healthy person facing west. By tapping this second person's abdomen, Dr. Abrams could not only diagnose the patient's illness but also tell his religion. Later he replaced this gizmo with the "oscillo-clast," a sort of souped-up dynamizer, which he manufactured and leased to other quacks.

This was the sort of heroic scale on which Brinkley longed to work. Somewhere, he thought, in the vast detritus of vibrometers, spectro-chrome pituitary stimulants, and foot-powered breast enlarg-ers lay the key.

5

At Fort Bliss, Texas, outside El Paso, First Lieutenant John R. Brinkley lay on his stomach in sick bay emitting sounds of anguish.

In the summer of 1917 the barbarians weren't anywhere near the gates, yet to his dismay he had been drafted anyway and sent here as doctor to the Sixty-fourth Infantry. As Brinkley later remembered it, the job was crushingly difficult: "I did the work ordinarily required of ten men. I had 2,208 raw recruits, without medical supplies, clothing or anything else. I was the only medical officer and worked day and night trying to get my troops vaccinated against typhoid and small pox, besides looking after the sanitation of the regiment. . . . My raw recruits were coming down with all kinds of infectious diseases like measles, meningitis, and besides I had to do the operating on those that needed surgery and treat those I had in quarters, visit my sick ones I had in the hospital, make out my technical reports and on top of all this, about twice a week I got orders every evening about six o'clock to be ready for debarkation the next morning. . . .

"When you take into consideration that one lone medical officer was doing all this work, it is no wonder that along in August I broke all to pieces and landed in the hospital." Upon his recovery, he said, he received "a surgeon's certificate of disability" and went on to render "private service to our government."

In fact, the record shows that of the two months and thirteen days he served in the army, Brinkley spent more than half the time in sick bay complaining of "rectal fistula, multiple." In August he got the boot.

Down to his last few dollars, he spotted a newspaper ad: Milford, Kansas, population two thousand, was looking for a doctor. He and Minnie loaded up their flivver and arrived there on October 7, 1917. On the edge of town Brinkley stopped, and the car shivered into silence. Milford had lied to them. Its population wasn't two thousand; it was two hundred, if it stood on a chair.

Located ninety-five miles north of Wichita and ten miles from the exact geographical center of the nation, Milford was about as close as you could get to the navel of the United States, and about as interesting to contemplate. In 1859 traveler Horace Greeley wrote that the buffalo moved quickly through the area, "as I should urgently advise them to do." Since then the town had grown to a length of two blocks. Its lone attempt at grandeur, a large building misguidedly salvaged from the 1904 St. Louis World's Fair, stood empty and derelict. The train station was in a cornfield.

Minnie took one look at Milford and burst into tears.

But they had no choice, so they rolled up their sleeves. The Brinkleys rented two rooms, opened an office in front, and put their iron bed in the back. They added a small drugstore. And in the weeks that followed they began to make a name for themselves. Brinkley traveled miles to make house calls, even after the snows hit, and Minnie hired out as a midwife. Even so, they were barely getting by.

Then one day a forty-six-year-old farmer, Bill Stittsworth, appeared at their door, big featured, unshaven, in a crumpled hat. His visit didn't seem like the Annunciation, any more than he looked like the archangel Gabriel. At least at first.

"There's something wrong with me," Stittsworth said when he'd taken a seat, "though to look at me you wouldn't judge it. I do look husky, don't I?"

Brinkley nodded and stroked his goatee, a habitual tic.

"I'm all in," the patient ventured. "No pep. I'm a flat tire."

Finally he spelled it out.

Dr. Brinkley (perhaps mindful he could be staying there a while) replied that over the years he had tried "serums, medicines and electricity," but nothing worked on that condition. There was no cure.

A pause as they gazed out the window.

"Too bad I don't have billy-goat nuts," the farmer remarked, pondering the livestock.

Exactly what happened next is in dispute. According to the book *Life of a Man* by Clement Wood, a self-promotional fantasia commissioned by Brinkley in the 1930s: "The doctor half closed his eyes and considered. . . . And then he shook his head, slowly. The code of ethics his father had drilled into him forever forbade him from any conduct, especially with relation to healing, except the utterly honest and straightforward."

The farmer pleaded and threatened. Brinkley demurred. What if something went wrong? But the patient wouldn't take no for an answer, and finally the doctor agreed to try.

That was his version. Stittsworth's family later contended that it was Brinkley who offered the farmer money, and then more money, hundreds of dollars, to submit to the experiment. However it happened, from Brinkley's point of view it was his ticket to the top—if it worked. He had always known that for an operator with big dreams the percentage of people with cancer, for example, is discouragingly small; but a working driveshaft is as fundamental as sunshine. What better place to hang out one's shingle?

Neither man wanted publicity, at least not yet, so two nights later while Milford slept, Stittsworth slipped back to the clinic. He stripped and climbed onto the operating table. Masked, gowned, and rubber gloved, Brinkley entered with a small silver tray, carried in both hands, like the Host. On it were two goat testicles in a bed of cotton. He set the tray down, injected anesthetic . . .

It was over in less than fifteen minutes. One of them paid the other and the farmer went home.

Days passed. The doctor's heart was a battleground of avarice and fear. Then, after two long weeks, the farmer reappeared with a smile on his face.

Now the goat was out of the bag. Stittsworth spread the word, and another farmer, age thirty-eight, tried it. Success! Other locals trickled in, like Charlie Tassine from the barbershop. Then Mrs. Stittsworth insisted on a matching set of goat ovaries.

"Dimly," wrote Clement Wood, "[Brinkley] had begun to realize that he was gifted beyond the run of doctors"—and that a man so blessed could not be bound by the "jealous sheep ethics" of the American Medical Association.

Some weeks later, Brinkley went to Chicago for a brush-up surgery course taught by Morris Fishbein's former professor, Dr. Max Thorek. Brinkley failed the class, as the teacher later explained, due to "his attendance not being regular, and because of his indulgence in alcohol. I admonished him to leave liquor alone and to concentrate on worthwhile endeavor and improve himself as a man and a physician, to which he replied, 'I have a scheme up my sleeve and the whole world will hear of it.'"

6

When he put farmer Stittsworth under the knife in November 1917, Brinkley became a pioneer in gland transplants. But he wasn't the only one. Buoyed by an ecstatic press and a handful of scientists with competing "breakthroughs," glandular "rejuvenation" was just dawning as an international craze. Whatever their differences, the top researchers agreed on this: they had stumbled on the greatest discovery in the history of mankind, a doorway not only to sexual strength but to the recovery of youth itself.

Good-bye, yogurt. For years Elie Metchnikoff, the 1908 Nobel Prize winner in physiology and medicine, had been flogging that as an antiage food, to the point where "it was the custom at directors' meetings," a Manhattan businessman said, "to reach into your pocket, take out your tube and take a drink of this concentrate in the belief that you were extending your life." Yale football coach Walter Camp had claimed the same for his "daily dozen" exercises. But when Metchnikoff and Camp both embarrassingly died before age seventy, it was time for some replacement magic, and this time it wouldn't be confined to a cult.

The notion of priming one's privates came naturally to the Jazz Age, as men and women chased bliss with a butterfly net after the horrors of the war. They swallowed things: royal jelly, for example, and "pega palo cocktails" derived from a plant called the vitality vine. For some there was more at stake than just a good party. The obliteration of millions of young men in battle, the cream of a generation, had left

31

Western society (especially Europe) with great gaps to fill, and in the short term older people would have to fill them. Instead of retiring, they would need to keep working and, if possible, breeding. Some saw it as a duty to their class, to prevent the offspring of degenerates and defectives from seizing the future of the white race. In short, the zeitgeist demanded the discovery of a way to recapture youth—first and foremost, male potency.

Only the urgency was new, not the dream. Ever since man began to walk upright, he had been obsessed when his penis would not behave likewise and searched for ways to fix the problem. The world's earliest-known medical document, the so-called Edwin Smith Papyrus of Egypt dating from 1600 B.C., presents a strikingly sophisticated view of trauma surgery—except on the back, where one finds "Incantation for Transforming an Old Man into a Youth of Twenty." In ancient Greece an herb called satyrion, recommended by the philosopher Theophrastus in 320 B.C., was swiftly harvested to extinction. During the ensuing centuries cloves, ginger, and massaging one's genitals in ass's milk all had their vogue. In England around the year 1000, men were devouring "love bread" (naked maidens romped in wheat, which was then harvested counterclockwise). The Middle Ages favored lubrication of the afflicted member with melted fat from camel humps.

Well, there would be no more of that silliness. Mankind had found wisdom at last. Science! Technology! These were the new church. Adam was out, apes were in. Rationality ruled. Rationality had made the airplane possible, and instant coffee. Few realized that it also made possible the golden age of quacks.

For as it turned out, the rush of scientific breakthroughs actually made people more credulous. Electricity at least made light you could see, but the twenties brought something called quantum physics, something else called sonar. Thanks to their astonishing new device, the thermocouple, Professors Pettit and Nicholson at the Mount Wilson Observatory in Pasadena were able to prove that Mars was fit for human habitation. Jackhammers! Atom smashing! In this dizzy world of wonders anything was possible, and it all conspired to make the average citizen as guileless as the wide-mouthed shad. One measure of the scientific gullibility of the age is the number of mythical animals that were now positively declared to exist. During this period between the world wars, sightings were reported and searches launched for, among others, the snoligostus, the ogopogo, the Australian bunyip, the whirling wimpus, the rubberado, the rackabore, and the cross-feathered snee.

Medical wonders got the same wild welcome. Strapping a metal contraption on one's head to cure stuffy nose, drinking radium as a cure for cancer, it all fit with the logic of modern life. Scientists themselves were the least skeptical of all. Breakthroughs in plastic surgery and orthopedics (largely due to the war) led British scientist Julian Huxley to foresee the day when "biological knowledge enable[s] us to modify the processes of our bodies more in accord with our wishes," and many of his fellow scientists thought that day could be soon, next year, next week. Advances in medicine and hygiene had already increased the average lifetime from forty-one years in 1870 to more than fifty-five by the early 1920s. Now the sky was the limit—biblical life spans, some researchers said, could become a reality—all thanks to the homely gonad and the brave new science of endocrinology.

What became the modern study of hormone-producing glands, or endocrines, began in the unsteady mind of Charles Edouard Brown-Sequard, a muttonchopped physiologist and former Harvard professor who, after a long and distinguished international career, wandered off the reservation in the late 1880s. Past seventy, "irritable, impotent, suffering from gastro-intestinal troubles and plagued by urinary disturbances" (as another doctor described him), he set up a small private lab in Paris and dropped from sight. But on June 1, 1889, he reemerged with a sensational speech before the Société de Biologie in which he claimed to have conquered Father Time by injecting himself with an emulsion of dog and guinea pig testicles. "All has changed," he declared, "and I have regained the full force that I possessed"—by which he meant both sexual potency and a "power of defecation" he had almost forgotten.

The reaction of his audience was a reported "uproar of incredulity and wrath." But the wider world was more receptive. The Paris newspaper *Le Matin* at once launched a subscription drive to found an institute of rejuvenation where clients could receive injections of the great *liquide testiculaire*. Within weeks a consortium of druggists announced a compound of their own called Spermine, consisting of "semen, calf's heart, calf's liver, bull's testicles," plus unspecified gleanings from "the surface of anatomical specimens kept under alcohol." Mixed together, they were said to give customers "the stimulant effects observed by Dr. Brown-Sequard." Other manufacturers launched similar products, but when scientists failed to replicate the professor's results, the market temporarily lost momentum.

However, though his work collapsed under scrutiny, Brown-Sequard's efforts were hardly a failure. Aside from making an army of quacks rich for decades to come, they also caught the fancy of legitimate scientists who believed—correctly—that there was something intuitively sound about his premise: that a key to enhanced vigor and muscle mass lurked somewhere in the secretions of the sex glands, if only they could figure out how to get at it. The professor's delusions thus became the source of the Nile for much of the sex-gland research in the decades ahead, leading to milestones like the isolation and synthesis of testosterone in the 1930s, and carrying right on through to doping with anabolic steroids. From the nut, Brown-Sequard, a mighty oak would grow.

Early on, however, in the first follow-ups to his work, scientists were as passionate as they were clueless. One hypothesis held that where Brown-Sequard went wrong was in using an emulsion; it wouldn't be strong enough. Perhaps if one manipulated the glands themselves . . . As experimentation picked up speed, rivalries among the top researchers turned fierce, leading to the first rush of competing "discoveries" around the time of the Great War.

Not long after joining the *Journal of the American Medical Asso-*

ciation, Morris Fishbein bumped into Dr. G. Frank Lydston on the street in Chicago. Professor of genitourinary surgery at the University of Illinois, Lydston was a scrappy character known for the rare breadth of his writings, which ranged from arcane technical works in his field to novels like *Poker Jim, Gentleman,* and *Over the Hookah.* "We chatted a moment," Fishbein recalled, "and then he said, 'Put your hand in here and feel.' He had opened his coat and shirt and he directed my hand to the side of his ribs. On each side I felt six or more nodules. I asked him what they were. 'Testicles,' he said. In an effort to rejuvenate himself he had transplanted under his skin testicular tissue obtained from bodies."

Since Brown-Sequard, most experiments had focused on transferring glands from one lower animal to another. But Lydston had made the great leap: he was the first to transplant testicles from one human to another. "With no thought of heroics," he wrote, "and impelled by the obvious practical facts, first that it was hardly fair to subject any one else to whatever dangers the experiment might involve, and second, that if I asked one of my professional friends to perform the operation I would lose the opportunity of being the pioneer in the field, I resolved to perform the operation upon myself." He thus became, as the *New York Times* phrased it, "this extraordinary trinity" of surgeon, patient, and clinical observer all in one.

Finding a donor—a challenge, one might have thought—was actually easy, thanks to the help of Dr. Leo Stanley, chief surgeon at San Quentin prison in California. Three or four hangings a year offered the perfect chance to relieve relatively young men of their testicles without an argument, and after the first operation on himself Lydston continued to experiment with convicts. Passed through an iced saline solution, testicles of deceased felons were inserted into other prisoners, usually geezers with no chance of parole. According to Dr. Stanley's reports, most showed improvement. Seventy-two-year-old Mark Williams, half-senile at the time of the implant, perked up within five days "and could even understand a joke."

The magnitude of the breakthrough, Lydston now claimed, went far beyond sexual performance. Not only had his own graying hair turned black again, he said, but he had found through his work with criminals that testicular implants retarded and even reversed senility. Scientific journals, including *JAMA*, gave his work wide and respectful coverage. Dr. Stanley himself, inspired by Lydston, plunged into experiments of his own and in the coming years injected or implanted testicular material, both animal and human, into 643 inmates and 13 physicians. He detailed his exhilarating findings in the journal *Endocrinology*. (Stanley had another, independent theory that physically unattractive people were more likely to become criminals—it was a way of revenging themselves on the world—so he also instituted a program of giving prisoners nose jobs.)

Though debunkers were heard loud and clear, claims like these sparked a sort of provisional joy in much of the Western world's scientific community. Dr. Max Thorek, who saw Lydston often in Chicago, said his "eagerness was so flaming as to amount to zealotry," and the same could be said of the two other great champions of glandular rejuvenation then taking the stage.

Like Lydston, they are unknown names today, not so much forgotten as scissored out of history or dropped down Orwell's memory hole. Other pioneer researchers of the day, like Pasteur and Madame Curie, are remembered as patron saints in their fields. But no practitioner of modern rejuvenation (life extension, practical immortality, it goes by different names now) wants portraits of the groundbreakers in his line hanging in the waiting room because these men were so deeply deluded that even to mention their theories now could turn a potential client into a fading scream. Nevertheless, great blunderers like these have a place in the history of science. Wrong, they helped point the way for others to be right. They fought as bravely for error as more fortunate prophets fought for the truth. In science, as in love, it is sometimes extraordinarily hard to draw the line between faith and folly.

Russian by birth, Dr. Serge Voronoff was a naturalized Frenchman based in Paris, where he served as director of the Laboratory of

Physiology at the Collège de France. A magnetic figure *"plus français que les français,"* as a friend said, Voronoff was six feet four, with a prowling imagination, and his interest in glands and longevity had been triggered as far back as 1898. Working in Egypt as attending physician to its ruler, Khedive Abbas II, he had treated some of the eunuchs attached to the king's harem. They were a fat and sickly lot. "The hair grows white at an early age," Voronoff wrote, "and it is rare for them to attain old age. . . . Are these disastrous effects directly due to the absence of the testicles?" If so, he reasoned, per-haps so-called normal aging was caused by the gonads wearing out—and a process so localized might thus be reversible.

He made tests. Early on he transplanted a lamb's testicles into an elderly ram and found, he said, that the ram's wool thickened and its sex drive reappeared. His researches interrupted by the Great War, Voronoff traveled extensively treating the wounded, devising "auto-grafts" using bone from the patients themselves (a technique others used successfully for decades), and replacing burned skin with fetal membrane. But the siren call of the animal kingdom soon reclaimed him, and this time it didn't come from a sheep.

"I dare assert," he declared after further experiments, "that the monkey is superior to man by the sturdiness of its body, the quality of its organs, and the absence of those defects, hereditary and acquired, with which the main part of mankind is afflicted."

His course was clear. In 1914 he first used a monkey as donor, grafting its thyroid gland into a "boy who was an idiot." The opera-tion reportedly went so well that soon "the boy was in a normal condition and found fit for the army." Voronoff was now certain that in the glands of the lower primates lay, if not eternal youth, something close to it. By his calculation monkey testicles should keep a man healthy and active for a century and a half, at which time he would simply collapse like the one-horse shay. All that remained was to nail down the proof.

Meanwhile rejuvenation's other great star, Dr. Eugen Steinach of Vienna, was pursuing his competing version of the grail. A professor at the Biological Institute, Steinach moved—along with Freud, Mahler, Reich, and Wittgenstein—in the city's most honored circles, a figure "of Jovian appearance," a colleague said, "with a luxuriant beard of superb Titian hue." Egotistical, touchy, with a smoldering paranoia that would worsen over time, he had a passion for horseback riding, a blood-red office, and the key to life—or so believed the many who pointed him out and applauded him on the street.

Compared with Voronoff's exotic construct, or Lydston's testicle packs, the Steinach method was simple. Experiments on rats led the Austrian to conclude that youth could be recovered by "ligation of the vas"—a vasectomy. Steinach theorized that the "secretions associated with ejaculation," dammed up, would flow backward throughout the body, creating a sort of masculine greenhouse effect. (Years later it was shown that unexpended semen is dissipated in the urine.) Like his rivals, he produced evidence ("Patient feels young, energetic, cheerful. In contrast to former years, he is now at the end of the theatre season, as fresh as he was at the beginning . . ."), including reports of hair growth, improved eyesight, and the curing of many diseases. And yes, it "raised the platform of efficiency" in faltering males. After triumphs in Europe, Steinach's name first surfaced professionally in the United States shortly after the war, when the *New York Medical Journal* called his work a "great advance" in combating senility.

Forever young! From the early 1920s to the late 1930s, throngs joined the great maypole dance around the human gland. Voronoff spoke for the entire movement when he wrote, in a book entitled simply *Life:* ". . . there is no doubt that the surgery of the future will consist largely in preserving and, when necessary, replacing the glands of the human body, in order to preserve life, vigor and health. . . .

"Does any scientific discovery of the ages exceed this in its importance to the individual and the race?"

7

In August 1918 John Brinkley opened a new sixteen-room clinic in Milford, Kansas. Called the Brinkley Institute of Health, it housed (according to his promotional pamphlet) the Brinkley-Jones Hospital, Brinkley-Jones Associates, the Brinkley Research Laboratories, and the Brinkley Training School for Nurses. Inside it looked less like a hospital than an overgrown bed-and-breakfast. The rooms were paneled in mahogany and Circassian walnut, the wallpaper was sky blue, and the townsfolk were delighted—not least the electrical contractor on the project who said that Brinkley "paid the best wages in the area."

His popularity was soaring. Not only was he a generous employer with a storybook marriage, bringing a swatch of eastern Kansas into financial bloom; the worldwide Spanish flu pandemic, the worst plague in history, had struck here, too, and Brinkley earned respect and gratitude that winter with his conspicuous efforts to help the victims. The doc "seemed to have an uncanny knack with the flu," one of his aides recalled. "Maybe it was something he learned as a boy in the North Carolina mountains. I don't know, but whatever it was, it worked." When more than a thousand cases broke out in nearby Fort Riley, Brinkley (in marked contrast to his imaginary exploits in the army) was on the spot helping to treat them. He went from farm to farm as well, bouncing along mud-rutted roads in a 1914 Ford. His driver, Tom Woodbury, remembered him as "a wonderful doctor. He lost only one patient during the flu epidemic and he doctored all around." A local housewife said, "He saved us. They called him a quack and that just breaks my heart. He was no quack, believe me."

When a coal shortage that winter made the suffering even worse, Brinkley led a petition drive demanding that the governor provide emergency allocations for flu victims. The entire performance, contrasted with the rest of his career, was so aberrant it is hard to credit. Maybe he was buying publicity. Maybe he had no choice. Whatever made Brinkley violate his charlatan code, the help he rendered during those months stands as the finest achievement of his life.

He soon righted himself and got back to goats, just as the first postwar surge of rejuvenation news was hitting the press. Although top-tier newspapers at first resolutely ignored him—while crying up Voronoff, Steinach, and Lydston—the man from Milford didn't seem to mind. He was too busy exploiting the respectability they enjoyed.

Déclassé or not, Dr. Brinkley nursed advantages over his rivals they never suspected: guile, marketing genius, and an inspired choice of animal. To most of his early clientele, farm folk from America's heartland, a goat's appetite for sex was famous. They had seen it all their lives. It was an archetype built into the language: *goatish* (horny, hot, lascivious). The ancient Greeks had Pan, half-goat, half-man, cavorting through glens and deflowering wood nymphs. Or go back even further, to the world's first known aphrodisiac recipe, recorded in the Buddhist text Samhita of Sushruta around the eighth century B.C. He who would "visit a hundred women," it said, should eat "the testes of a goat, either by boiling the testes in milk and adding sesame seeds and lard of a porpoise, or by mixing the testes with salt, powdered pepper fish and clarified butter." All of this lurked in the human subconscious, part of the luggage Brinkley's patients toted to his Kansas clinic, along with their sacrificial goats and their $750 cash, no credit, no exceptions.

Soon after his clinic opened, Brinkley scored a publicity coup big enough to bring the first big-city reporters to his door: Mrs. Stittsworth, wife of Brinkley's first gland patient, gave birth to a bouncing baby boy—named Billy, perhaps after the goat. A news photo of the doctor and the infant smiling together for the camera carried the caption: "Dr. John R. Brinkley, a surgeon, has startled the scientific world by transplanting goat glands to men and women as a means of restoring a lost heritage." When that got around, a wave of new female clients overwhelmed the town, pitching tents in Milford's groves and pastures. Thanks to the intrepid Mrs. Stittsworth and her pioneering goat ovaries, Brinkley started a side business in that line, promoting them as a fertility enhancer, wrinkle reducer, and bust developer.

As for the benefits of the goat testicle, he claimed they had scarcely been tapped. Letters from former patients reported an "astonishing sexual vigor" whose details "cannot be more than hinted at." And there was more good news, Brinkley said, citing the case of a deranged youth who

> had been told finally that he was incurable and must remain a mental defective. He had decided to commit suicide if I failed to remedy his condition.
>
> In 36 hours after the insertion of goat glands this patient's temperature had risen to above 103°F. but became normal twenty-four hours later, and has since remained so. His mind has gradually cleared, he looks and feels younger and is contemplating marriage. The hideous dreams and nightmares which had destroyed his sleep and rest all his past life have left him. . . .
>
> My second case of insanity [caused this time by excessive masturbation] was a young bank clerk brought to me from a state institution. Following gland transplantation, his mind cleared completely and he is now head of a large banking institution.

Curing sexual problems and dementia praecox was only the beginning. The "Ponce de León of Kansas" soon discovered that goat glands worked wonders on twenty-seven different ailments big and small, from emphysema to flatulence. Brinkley cautioned that there were no guarantees; his operation only had about a 95 percent success rate. He added cannily that it worked less well on "stupid types."

This put him for the first time on the radar of the AMA. Always suspicious of stratospheric claims, it sent a private detective to visit the clinic undercover. There he met a woman in her sixties, partially paralyzed. Brinkley had given her goat ovaries to treat a spinal cord tumor. "She seemed to hobble along, dragging one foot after the other," the agent reported. "I assisted the old lady from one room to the other, she wanted to demonstrate how she could walk. She shuffled along very slowly and stated that she felt like she had a little more action in her legs."

But Brinkley's bread and butter was still impotent men, and as business grew he set up a shuttle service to meet them at the train. When they arrived at the depot, usually on Monday afternoons, bus driver Happy Harry was there to greet them with his chauffeur's cap atilt and a twinkle in his eye. They already knew about Harry from the form letters the doc mailed out. They knew about Minnie, too: "If Mrs. Brinkley lived near you, she would share with you the choicest flowers from her yard, the nicest 'roastin' ears' from her garden. She would run over to your house on Sunday with a big pail of homemade ice cream that she thought was specially good." And when they climbed out of the van, there she was, Minnie in person, standing in the doorway of the clinic with her cookie maker's smile: "Here come my men."

The new arrivals were slippered and gowned in the "herd room." Then came their first audience with the doctor himself, which usually cemented their faith. A portrait photo of Brinkley from this period shows a smallish gentleman wearing round, rubber-rimmed glasses and chin whiskers (echoing the goat). Head to the side, he has the look of a man prepared for some intellectual ping-pong, perhaps with Europeans. Add to this his signature slogans—"All energy is sex energy" and "A man is as old as his glands"—and you had the perfect road-company Freud. Nor was it all a sham. Brinkley's uncanny grasp of psychology, both mass and individual, was a vital part of his success. He understood that the relationship between a man and a woman is often less fraught than that between man and member, and his skill in exploiting that knowledge ranks among his greatest gifts.

Of course he hit the occasional snag. One day a couple of adventurous swells arrived from California to receive new glands. Although

Brinkley had settled on Toggenburg goats as best for his purposes, they insisted on Angora, a tonier breed. Too late they discovered it left their genitals with an eye-opening aroma.

But mostly the doctor piled one triumph on the next. A second goat gland baby was born to a Milford businessman and his wife. They named him Charles Darwin Mellinger, in honor of science. At Christmastime, Dr. and Mrs. Brinkley climbed onto the roof of their clinic and threw oven-ready turkeys, geese, and ducks into the outstretched arms of their neighbors.

It was all so friendly, so deeply communal. Is it possible that, like Steinach and Voronoff and Lydston, Brinkley believed in what he was doing?

The answer lies perhaps in small things, like his way of calling patients "old fools" when he was drunk. Or perhaps in larger things, like his wavering conception of what a goat-gland transplant actually was. Sometimes he slivered the animal gland like a clove of garlic and put the pieces in the patient. Sometimes he joined the smaller testicle to the larger, a process he likened to "embedding a marble in an apple." Sometimes the operation was no more complex than tossing a Christmas present into a bag. Skill wasn't the issue—technically speaking, he was a competent surgeon when he put his mind to it— but quality control was iffy at best. Brinkley performed operations both before and after the cocktail hour, and as his enterprise expanded he passed off more and more of the work to assistants with medical credentials even wispier than his own. As a result dozens of patients died over the years, either in the operating room or shortly after their return home. Many others were permanently maimed. Still it would be a long time before anyone equated his clinic with wholesale murder. Meanwhile, whatever the outcome, Brinkley expected to be paid.

By early 1920 there were rumors he was stealing goats from neighboring farms when he ran short. In the meantime, hoping to grow the business even faster, the doctor sought advice from a professional adman. That brought H. Roy Mosnat of Kansas City to his door. Surprisingly, Mosnat seems to have arrived knowing nothing about Brinkley's practice—at least that's how they both remembered it—but the moment he heard he leapt to his feet in delight.

"By God, we've got it! Dr. Brinkley, you've got a million dollars within your hands!"

On the drive out to Stittsworth's farm, Mosnat gazed at the world like a man in love. ("There were white masses of clouds floating up there in the blue . . .") He and Stittsworth had a conference by the pump and then, his pockets stuffed with notes, Mosnat caught the next train back to Kansas City to map his campaign.

It was a fateful moment, for even more than the goat-gland racket itself, it was the doctor's determination to advertise that put him on a collision course with the AMA. The organization had forbidden any advertising by its members (Brinkley then was one) even before Samuel Hopkins Adams's series in *Collier's,* but the policy turned even more strict after it appeared. One of Adams's revelations was that patent medicines provided as much as half the ad revenue taken in by America's newspapers, a corrupt alliance of vast proportions. Ads were routinely tarted up to look like news. Even when they weren't, they were preposterous and offensive, from the woodcuts of people shooting themselves through the head ("the result of neglected nervousness") to noisome appeals to patriotism, like the full-page representation of Uncle Sam signing a scroll: "This is to certify that I am using 100,000 boxes of Ex-Lax every month." Such was the marriage of "health" and marketing, and respectable doctors shunned it like the devil himself.

When Brinkley started advertising, then, he made a formal enemy of the AMA. As it happened, the doctor didn't like Mosnat's work. He thought it too tame, especially when only two reporters in the country wrote new stories about him.

But it was enough.

8

In June 1920, Dr. Max Thorek, chief surgeon at the American Hospital in Chicago, bumped into Dr. Frank Lydston in an elevator. Lydston had an office in the building.

"Have you got a moment to spare, Max?" he asked. Thorek later described what happened next:

"We entered his office and without any explanation, as soon as we were behind locked doors, he began to disrobe. I was annoyed and puzzled. Suddenly, he turned around, as nude as a classic statue of Apollo. . . .

"'Take a look.'

"A physician learns not to be surprised, but on this occasion I was overwhelmed with amazement. . . . Lydston had three testicles."

Not content with the implants to his abdominal wall, the University of Illinois professor had raised the experimental bar, adding the gonad of an executed prisoner to his own. Three balls gave the best results yet, he declared. It had boosted both his sex drive and the speed and clarity of his thinking—and no, taking a murderer's testicle on board had not given him criminal impulses. Thorek, a leathery old skeptic more interested in amateur photography than glands, listened to Lydston, saw his messianic glow—and began to believe. He sat rapt while Lydston talked for three hours.

During this spiel the Hungarian began to sense something else, a sort of nervous rage simmering beneath Lydston's excitement. Just days before, on June 12, Dr. Serge Voronoff had made international news with the first monkey-to-man testicle transplant. Lydston believed that Voronoff had stolen from his own work (which had been published in *JAMA*) and was getting the attention he himself deserved, while taking the less challenging course of using monkeys. This made Thorek begin to wonder if Lydston's impulsive third testicle was more a stroke of one-upmanship than a scientific advance.

Thorek was sympathetic to Lydston's viewpoint, but he felt a higher loyalty to the truth. He left at once for New York, where Voronoff was scheduled to give his first American demonstration. There, before a distinguished host at Columbia University's College of Physicians and Surgeons, the Russian proudly—in English, with an oddly French accent—unveiled his technique. Thorek became convinced that Voronoff, not Lydston, was on the right track, and he invited the Russian to Chicago to repeat the demonstration.

Voronoff had that generosity of spirit, that refusal to see the world in terms of winners and losers, that often makes winners so obnoxious. No sooner had he arrived in Chicago than he paid a courtesy call to Dr. Lydston's laboratory. When he learned what the American had been working on lately, Voronoff reportedly cried out, "Oh, zat is fine! Your operations are for zee poor man and mine are for zee rich man!"

Lydston was beside himself. Not only was this credit grabber right there in his own office, peering at labels and opening drawers, but the treacherous Dr. Thorek had brought him to town to put on a show. As Lydston feared, it was the event of the year. "What a day that was for us—for all the profession in Chicago!" Thorek wrote. "Every inch of the amphitheater in our hospital was crowded. Notables were scattered everywhere throughout the audience." Assisted like a stage magician by his young and beautiful American wife, Voronoff dazzled the hall with a lecture-demonstration using dogs. Only two important people were missing from the audience. One was Lydston, who—until his death soon after at age sixty-five—never forgave Voronoff for stealing his thunder. The other was John Brinkley, who tried to crash the party. Dr. Thorek spotted him, however, and barred his "slimy" former student at the door.

But Brinkley hadn't wasted a trip. Mosnat, the adman, had generated enough heat to get the goat-gland surgeon an important invitation to Park Avenue Hospital in Chicago to prove what he could do. Thus did three of rejuvenation's stars converge that summer of 1920, igniting the craze in earnest and setting the stage for the "Milford Messiah" to become the biggest star of all.

Recently the doctor had been refining his message. Ever since the birth of little Billy Stittsworth, Brinkley had often described his mission as helping desperate women to conceive ("Dr. J. R. Brinkley Swamped with Letters from Women Craving Halo of Motherhood"). Responding to these bags of mail—"I would give my life if I could bring a baby into the world," one woman wrote—Brinkley said he was "overwhelmed" by their "heartbreaking" pleas, and considered himself blessed to be able to help so many in this plight, especially since his discovery that hysterectomies could be reversed by implanting ovaries from a goat.

By mid-1920, however, Brinkley was drifting off this claim—the breast-enlarging and wrinkle-reducing parts, too—to concentrate on his male clientele, having found perhaps that women had a narrower eye for results. From here on, heirs would be incidental; transforming the bedroom bumbler into "the ram that am with every lamb" was his top selling point. With men he could ride the placebo effect like an elephant. In fact, men would apparently believe anything, like the one who wrote to ask if goat glands would help his sex life after he'd twice been struck by lightning.

Brinkley's lucky appearance in Chicago that summer in company with his rivals gave him a new luster of respectability. Indeed, it enabled him to steal the inside track, for while the others were conscientiously mired in demonstrations and experiments, and documenting their progress in scientific journals, he could skip all that and go right to work helping suffering humanity.

The believers who flocked to him came from all walks of life, not just the farm or laboring classes. Meditating on the inexhaustible theme of human credulity, a British medical writer of the time observed: "It is commonly said that education is a great safeguard against quackery and faddery. I profoundly disbelieve it. So far as I can see, the higher one goes in the social scale, the more does fashion in health matters prevail, and the so-called *intelligentsia* are the most gullible of all."

So it proved at the Park Avenue Hospital in Chicago that summer, where Brinkley performed thirty-four goat-gland transplants (thirty-one of them male; subjects including a judge, an alderman, a society matron), pausing often to chat with reporters. He was pleased, he said, that Europeans had "accepted" gland work, though in candor he had to say that his own technique, in which the goat gland "humanized" in the scrotal sac, was "far in advance of the Old World experts." With Lydston on the ragged edge, reporters were only too glad to promote America's other, less crazed major player. His first Chicago clients were barely out of surgery when the cheering started: "The operations, whereby youth has been restored to the aged patients and vigor revived, were performed by Dr. J. R. Brinkley. . . . Their success has inundated him with business." Thanks to the surgical swami from Kansas, Chicagoans had "found the Lost Fountain of Youth."

One testimonial in particular made the Milford Messiah a national star. It came from seventy-one-year-old J. J. Tobias, chancellor of the University of Chicago Law School, who was described by the *Syracuse Herald* as "a thin, small, wiry type, incredibly frolicsome" with a crushing handshake. After the operation, did he really feel younger?

"I feel twenty-five years younger," the chancellor cried. "I am a new man, full of pep, strong, healthy, ready to go on with my work. I was ill, old and played out, but the operation has revivified me."

He dropped into a put-'em-up boxer's pose.

"How does it feel to have been old," the reporter asked, "and then be young again?"

"Glorious! . . . It is so wonderful it is almost unbelievable. The public cannot appreciate what the operation means. There has been some levity over the news of gland operations, but they should be treated with the greatest respect and admiration."

The hosannas of the law-school administrator were accompanied by a newspaper photo that showed him clicking his heels in midair, a shot so irresistible it was reprinted from coast to coast.

Not everyone was so infatuated with Dr. Brinkley's work. The health department didn't like his stabling fifteen goats at the hospital in August, and there was a startling burst of anger from the Chicago Federation of Labor. At their summer meeting Brinkley was denounced as anti-workingman: "These operations will increase the birth rate in the United States, and this increase will be a benefit to employers, and a detriment to union labor and higher wages."

Meanwhile, Max Thorek was excoriating Brinkley at every turn. Goat-gland transplants were not only "blasphemous, pornographic and obscene," the Hungarian declared, but "a physical and physiological impossibility resorted to only by the unscrupulous, who prey on the credulity of the public."

Monkeys on the other hand . . . After Voronoff left town, Dr. Thorek assembled an experimental zoo on the roof of the American Hospital to pursue gland experiments of his own. A menagerie of white rats, guinea pigs, rabbits, dogs, rhesus monkeys, baboons, and two chimpanzees was caged among bins of carrots, turnips, bananas, potatoes, oranges, coconuts, and hay. Abandoning most of his surgical practice, Thorek practically lived there. "My investment grew until thousands of dollars had gone to the apes. . . . I passed my days and nights with the animals.

"Was the ancient mystery of rejuvenation to be penetrated by the twentieth century? I knew that the quest of rejuvenation had long been a jack-o'-lantern, leading other investigators astray."

9

Audacity, more audacity, always audacity . . .

Brinkley stoked the publicity furnace hard after Chicago, and in some quarters his name took on a supernatural glow. During a tour of New England in the summer of 1921, the goat-gland king referred to other experiments he was engaged in that promised equally breathtaking benefits—his success transplanting eyes, for example, from one animal species to another. "At this moment I cannot [cure the blind]," he told an audience of Connecticut doctors. "Six months from now I think I will be able to." No evidence exists that he ever performed such experiments; he never mentioned them again, but the claim alone served its purpose. There were whispers that soon he might be able to raise the dead.

Back in Milford, the gland business practically ran itself. Gone was the chaos of patients dragging in their own goats. Now an Arkansas supplier delivered regular shipments of forty. The doctor kept them in a pen behind the clinic. Each client was invited to browse the herd and choose the most simpatico.

Those who worked for Brinkley, even those nearest him, still found him a hard man to figure. He could twirl a six-gun like a cowboy star, and sometimes liked to prove it, but he usually came across as a sort of down-home egghead, crisply confident and alert to a thousand details. Now and then he turned opaque, perhaps even shy. (One longtime staffer actually claimed he was "uncomfortable meeting people for the first time.") It was hard to get him on the telephone, and sometimes at the clinic he would vanish for portions of the day—partly, he told his aide Dr. Osborn, to get more done, and partly to cultivate his mystique. "You must get yourself so organized that people can't find you and see you to talk with you," he advised. Besides, he "never thought talking to people helped them get well."

The high whine of energy that drove him stayed mostly concealed. One night, though, he got liquored up and demolished a neighbor's car with an ax. Another time patients were seen bursting out of the hospital into the back garden, followed an instant later by Brinkley, drunk again and waving a butcher knife. In March 1921 a Milford resident named Jesse Wilson had a protection order taken out against him. As Brinkley explained it, "I made some remarks concerning this fellow that caused him to be afraid, I guess, and they put me under a bond; I don't know whether I was arrested or not, but I had to give a bond [of $1,000] not to shoot him."

Around town it was widely believed he had chewed off poor Osborn's ear.

Still, most of the locals were willing to view these shenanigans as the eccentricities of genius, since, thanks to him, Milford was rolling in dough. Along with a new, even larger hospital, Brinkley funded new sidewalks, a new municipal sewer system, a new post office, and new uniforms for the Little League team, now called the Brinkley Goats. He gave the town electric lights and a new bank. He paved the two-mile road to the railroad station, and he bought a bear in a failed attempt to start a zoo. (The bear's bellowing kept him awake at night, so he shot it.) Only once did the townsfolk balk at his generosity: when he tried to name the new church after himself. The way he saw it, a resident recalled, "Christ did not build the Milford Church; therefore it would not bear Christ's name, but would be called the Brinkley Methodist Church." The doctor had to settle for a plaque on the building honoring God, Jesus, and himself, along with this delirious tribute from the pastor: "You are possessed with power, unlike anything I ever found in any man before, and it affects me strangely. It caused me one Sunday to rush from your presence to the radio and say things I never knew I said. The critics said I likened you to Jesus of Nazareth. . . . I said I felt I had come from His presence. When you sit there on your exalted plane, you inspire me."

Lurching from one celebration to the next, the town became a virtual bacchanal of ice-cream socials and civic pride. "On Monday morning at 10 a.m.," the local paper reported, "a crowd collected at the Methodist church and marched with flags in hand, led by Walter Tague, to the park where a crowd was waiting. . . . A tribute to the flag was given by Dr. J. R. Brinkley. The national anthem was sung by all." The whole town threw Minnie a birthday party. And Brinkley promised even greater wonders to come, including a new hospital-cum-department-store modeled on the White House: "It will cover a whole block, will cost me a million dollars, and have shops, stores, a gymnasium, a monster bathing pool, beauty parlors, rooms for my clinic, and a theatre almost as big as the Orpheum in Kansas City, where we will give the best theatrical shows and talking pictures."

Until then the real Orpheum would have to do.

He was on a pleasure trip to Kansas City, tipped back in a barber's chair, when he noticed a man putting on his collar in front of the mirror. It was a deft performance considering the man had only one arm.

Brinkley sent the porter over, and James Crawford felt a tap on his shoulder. As he described their reunion, "[Brinkley] asked me how I was getting along and I told him, 'Very well,' and he informed me that he was running a hospital in a little town in Kansas—Milford, Kansas. . . . He said he was making considerable money and that he was getting along fine and I asked him if he was running this hospital on the order that we ran our office and he said, 'Very similar,' or words to that effect."

The doctor didn't elaborate. Such modesty was uncharacteristic, but no doubt he was wary of sharing the full facts: that he was now averaging fifty operations a month at $750 apiece, for a take of almost half a million dollars a year (in 1920s currency). Most patients walked in and lay down without even asking how the thing worked. "I suppose a goat gland is a good deal like a potato," said seventy-seven-year-old A. B. Pierce of Nebraska. "You can cut a potato all in pieces and plant it and every eye will grow."

Brinkley also had another quiet income stream, one inspired by Dr. Lydston. The Ponce de León of Kansas performed the occasional human-to-human testicle transplant, marketing it as the procedure of choice for those accustomed to large homes and fine wines.

It was a rich man's game, no question. Stories had surfaced over the past year or two of impoverished young men offering one of their testicles for sale, and other reports, even more unsettling, of youths kidnapped and castrated to supply the wealthy and depraved. Compared with predators like these, Brinkley was a paragon of ethics: his merchandise came strictly from death row. An Oklahoma oilman, for example, who wrote the doctor asking about goat glands (both for himself and some friends) received this reply:

> You are able to pay the full price for the boon of youth
> fully restored—why not do so? Why lower yourself to
> the level of the beasts of the field by having the glands
> of a goat transplanted into your body, when you may
> just as well have the glands of a healthy young man
> implanted in you?
>
> I will do this for you. If each of your friends come
> at the same time and will pay $5,000 each for a genuine
> human gland operation, I will give you the same kind of
> human gland operation which I perform at a minimum
> fee of $5,000. I have just closed with a case in Los
> Angeles today for $10,000. Few surgeons can get
> human glands, but I have an old-time friend in one
> of our large cities that can supply me.

Of course, these human gland operations are expensive. I pay a big price for the glands. I must have advance notice. For instance, if you and your friends decide to do this, you must notify me that you will be ready to leave any time within the next six weeks. Then I notify my purchasing agent and he gets busy. He may get the glands in a few days or he may wait weeks. So, it's necessary for my patients to be ready to come here when I am ready, and a cash payment of at least one-fourth must be sent me as a deposit so that I will not go and contract for something and be the loser.

I guarantee the human glands pure and healthy and absolutely free from disease. I also guarantee that the seller of them will not be over 35 years of age, thus insuring strong, virile glands.

Furthermore, I give another, and the best of all guarantees, that the human glands will not slough; if they do I will replace them free of charge within sixty days after the first operation, the patient only paying our regular hospital fees.

This deluxe option was little known to the wider world. Certainly not to Crawford, who disappeared again from Brinkley's life—for a time.

How did the doctor handle all this success? At the end of yet another long day, he was unwinding in a first-floor room of his clinic with some bootleg hooch, in company with several staffers. The talk grew lively, the liquor flowed, till suddenly Brinkley lunged for the instrument case, announcing he was going to "cut all their throats." Nurses tried to hold him, but he wrenched free and gave his visiting father-in-law, Dr. Tiberius Gracchus Jones, a severe bite wound on the thumb.

Hearing the shouts and crashes from below, patients on the second floor became alarmed. One leapt from his bed, knotted some sheets together, and started to lower himself out the window trying to run away. Before he reached the ground, however, he paused against the side of the building, ear cocked to the sudden silence. Brinkley's assistant, Dr. Osborn, had brought matters to a close by clubbing his boss over the head with a board.

10

In February 1922 the doctor received a brusque invitation from Harry Chandler, owner of the *Los Angeles Times,* to come to the West Coast and put goat glands in one of his editors. "If the operation is a success," Chandler wrote, "I'll make you the most famous surgeon in America. If it's a failure, I'll damn you with the same gusto." The doctor—one of the most famous surgeons in America already—didn't think twice.

He slid into Los Angeles like a duck onto a new pond, perfectly at home. The city's main boulevard had just been named for real-estate speculator and "magnetic-belt" quack Gaylord Wilshire, known around town by his medicine man's Vandyke, loud waistcoat, and checkered pants. In fact, with a population of roughly six hundred thousand, the Wonder City was viewed by many experts (Morris Fishbein included) as the most quack-intensive town in the nation. Local author Mayo Morrow promised that "any wizard, geomancer, soothsayer, holy jumper, herb doctor, whirling dervish, snake charmer, medicaster, table turner or Evil Eye, practicing any form of black magic, demonology, joint jerking, witchcraft, thaumaturgy, spirit rapping, back rubbing, physical torture or diabetical novelty . . . will find assured success and prosperity in Los Angeles despite fierce competition." A visitor from New York discovered whole buildings "devoted to occult and outlandish orders" whose leaders "fill the papers with mystic balderdash. They parade the streets in plush kimonos. . . . They dangle the tinsel star of erudition before the eyes of the semi-educated."

Not only were charlatans found here in tropical profusion, but the vast sucker pool was made up in large part of the sort of people Brinkley already knew well. Thousands of retirees and fresh starters had come here from America's midsection, ex-grocers, hardware merchants, hairdressers, farmers, half-exhausted men and women who had saved a little money or sold the old homestead and wanted to see the ocean before they died. They lived in small bungalows with a palm or banana tree out front, organized culture clubs and parades to march in, puttered in the garden—and sat. To many the boredom came as a shock. Paradise wasn't supposed to be dull. With minds cast adrift by the climate, the orange blossoms and heliotrope, many of these lifelong puritans turned naturally to God. But God wore different duds out here, like everybody else.

Dr. Leon Tucker with the Musical Messengers in a Great Bible Conference. 3 Meetings Tomorrow. Organ Chimes, Giant Marimbaphone, Vibraphone, Violin, Piano, Accordeon [sic], Banjo, Guitar and Other Instruments. Wilshire Baptist Church

Miss Leila Castberg of the Church of Divine Power (Advanced Thought)

Hear 10 Evangelists—10

N.C. Beskin, the CONVERTED Jew, back from a successful tour, will conduct a tabernacle campaign in Glendale. WHY I BECAME A CHRISTIAN. Dressed in Jewish garb. Will exhibit interesting paraphernalia

And these were the Sunday morning services. Elsewhere, in sanctified walk-ups and aromatic dens, far stranger tours of the spirit world were on sale seven days a week, and thousands threw off decades of straitlaced monotony to line up for them.

The other great void filler was fussing about one's health. Quite a few of these midwestern immigrants had come to California in the first place to ease their bones in the sun, and as more and more of the rest grew tired of bingo, it was no surprise that the most often-heard question after "Where do you come from?" was "How do you feel?" These people, who had pulled up stakes and traveled far to get here, were hopers by definition. Add it all up and you had the greatest flock of pigeons ever assembled.

But first things first. Brinkley went to see Harry Chandler and made arrangements to install goat glands in his employee. Chandler was a dynamo himself. Tall, in his late fifties, he had been so cherubically photogenic as a boy that his photo had been used to sell picture frames. But while he still wore the soft ghost of that face, behind it lay a rapacity of monumental proportions. He was "southern California's modern Midas," a man who invested in everything from oil to aircraft to the emerging tourist industry. The goal of his Yosemite National Park Company was to build shopping centers and hotels there. ("A lot of people complain that there is not much to do except look at the scenery and camp," one company official explained. "We are going to give the people what they want.") Primarily, though, Chandler bought and sold land, compulsively and insatiably: a million and a half acres of prime southern California real estate over the years. He earned one hundred million dollars orchestrating the notorious Owens River project, which took the water of valley farmers and sluiced it into Los Angeles, fostering the construction boom that created the modern city. (Noah Cross, the John Huston character in *Chinatown*, was partially based on Chandler.) Prior to that he had tried to seize part of Mexico by sending a private army against Pancho Villa. Indicted for "attempting to organize an insurrection" against a foreign power, Chandler was tried by a jury of his peers—prominent *Los Angeles Times* advertisers—and found not guilty.

His newspaper, most agreed, was lousy.

Brinkley and Chandler got along fine. Though the doctor had

licenses to practice in twelve states, California wasn't one of them, so the publisher pulled a string or two and got him a thirty-day permit. Brinkley applied for a permanent license as well and then began work that, as a visiting authority, he explained with rare precision: "Laboratory analysis shows that a goat gland contains 89 and 9/10ths percent ionized matter in a colloidal state; that it throws off emanations like radium; that it contains three princip[al] rays, alpha, beta and gamma; that it is capable of producing hormonie, which is thrown into the bloodstream." Basing himself at the Alexandria Hotel, he operated first on managing editor Harry E. Andrews. Success was proclaimed on March 23, 1922. Then the doctor did the same for a U.S. circuit court judge, unnamed Hollywood screen stars, and others. According to several reports, Chandler received goat glands himself.

> **New Life In Glands—Dr. Brinkley's Patients Here
> Show Improvement—Many Victims Of "Incurable"
> Diseases Are Cured—Twelve Hundred Operations
> Are All Successful**
> —*Los Angeles Times,* April 9, 1922

Brinkley cleared forty thousand dollars, Chandler cheered him to the skies, and when the testimonials began appearing, they claimed the expected multiple benefits. One California man wrote to thank the doctor for his new glands, "the swelling of the body having disappeared, and the drooling being much less." Buster Keaton put goat-gland gags in his new two-reeler, *Cops,* a publicity coup in itself.

In his spare time Brinkley explored Los Angeles. He was enchanted. After dark, spotlights raked the sky, electric signs blazed— 2,000,000 POPULATION BY 1930—and the movie palaces and posh dance halls were dressed to kill in neon. Pleasure and prosperity ("untempered," Aldous Huxley noted, "by any mental sauce") had swept into town along with the water from the Owens River spillway. Quacks were a force in local politics: AMA-backed efforts to require vaccines, quarantines, even a rabies muzzle law for dogs, had all been beaten back. In a word, it was Eden.

Harry Chandler was in the midst of constructing Los Angeles's first radio station, KHJ. Brinkley saw it and had a religious experience. Then the chamber of commerce offered to build their distinguished visitor a hundred-thousand-dollar hospital if he would settle there. He began at once to look for a site.

This wasn't the first time he had tried to relocate. Two years before, during his great summer of success, Brinkley had made ambitious plans to leave Milford for Chicago. "What we plan will, in fact, be a new school of medicine," he announced on August 5, 1920. "The course of instruction probably will cover four years. None should get the idea that the transplanting of animal glands can be taught in a few weeks. That is only part of the work." He had done what he could for Milford, he said, but he could no longer afford to carry the whole town on his shoulders.

Up till then the medical establishment had more or less quietly viewed him with revulsion, but this was too much. Prominent Chicago doctors attacked him in concert. Not only was the goat-gland operation a fake, but Brinkley didn't even have a license to practice in Illinois. Look at his credentials: before he started a medical school, he should graduate from a real one himself. That he had just been declared a doctor of science by the Chicago Law School—a strange honorary degree engineered by J. J. Tobias—hardly sufficed.

But the finishing blow to Brinkley's hopes came straight from the American Medical Association. Amid all the swooning over glands European and otherwise, the AMA had been a leading (if largely unheeded) voice of caution. Editorials in *JAMA* withheld judgment on glandular rejuvenation, calling for more studies and warning against "the ease at which fragmentary data are woven into a story of technical success." Morris Fishbein was especially skeptical, asserting that "far more proof is necessary before even a hope can be offered that a method of rejuvenation has been found." The use of goat glands he regarded as laughable, and Dr. Arthur Dean Bevan, onetime president of the AMA, called Brinkley's claims "rot."

So he'd been chased out of Chicago. But how fortunate after all! To set up shop in enemy territory, in the very shadow of AMA headquarters, would have been asking for trouble anyway. Far wiser to relocate half a continent away, with a buffer zone of warring medical boards and a thousand noisy newspapers. The air in California sweetly recommended itself; more to the point, he could make more money here. Brinkley spent several weeks looking for the right location—it was like choosing from a box of chocolates—before settling on a site: the Hidalgo Hotel in Ensenada. On June 18 he announced he would convert it into a thirty-six-room hospital. "I secured a location at Ensenada because of what appear to be climatic conditions peculiarly favorable to goat-gland operations," he said. "To perform the operation most successfully the surgeon should be located where the climate ranges around 70 degrees and is not subject to sharp changes. . . . If the undertaking proves successful a group of Los Angeles business men stand ready to erect there an institution to cost from $500,000 to $1,000,000." (With Brinkley there was always a dream behind the dream; it's sometimes hard to know for sure which he really nursed, and which were simply magic clouds of advertising.) He promised a facility run "along the lines of the Battle Creek health resort," with the bonus of goat glands. The animals would be supplied by a rancher in Del Monte.

Back in Chicago, things played out as the doctor had expected—almost. Generally speaking, the leadership of the AMA was happy to forget him as long as he was out of sight. But one member of the medical establishment wouldn't let go. Morris Fishbein retained pungent memories of Brinkley from the goat-gland demonstrations in Chicago two years before. Now, goaded by the ballyhoo coming out of L.A., the editor went to work. It would grow, stage by stage, into the greatest cause of his career: the professional extermination of John Brinkley, M.D.

11

In August 1922, while Brinkley awaited approval from the California licensing board, Sinclair Lewis sat at the desk in his room at Chicago's Morrison Hotel. Still riding the acclaim for *Main Street,* his corrosive novel of small-town life, Lewis was writing a letter to his wife, Grace, to tell her about an extraordinary person he had just met: "Fishbein is a wonder! Science, logic, immense knowledge not only of medicine . . . but of history—literature—a hundred things, humor, generous & eager interest. . . . [He is] opening up new worlds—& smashing bad old ones with relentless knowledge & sanity."

He had that effect on people. Buoyant, compulsively curious, Fishbein seemed at times like a modern Mr. Pickwick, if that gentleman had trained in medicine and marinated in the borscht belt for some years. His roaring energy, however, more closely recalled Dickens himself. On the golf course Fishbein played gin rummy between strokes. The murder trial of Leopold and Loeb so enthralled him, he advised both the prosecution and the defense. There were those who on first meeting him felt a strong impulse to back out of the room, but most were drawn to this rare individual who for better or worse (since past a point his strengths became limitations) seemed to exist almost entirely in the present tense.

Lewis liked something else about him, too, as the letter went on to explain. The day before there had been an unexpected knock at the door, and "in come Dr. Morris Fishbein, Carl Sandburg, & Harry Hansen & Keith Preston, literary editors of the Chi Daily News, AND Morris has Something [bootleg whiskey] in a grave-looking MS bag, and

I phone down [to] Room Service for White Rock, cracked ice, & 5 thin glasses. . . . And bimeby we all go out to dinner, & down to Fishbein's flat for an evening of great talk; & I stay overnight; & here I am back."

Their friendship had launched with Fishbein's warm review of Lewis's novel in the *Chicago Daily News*. ("For the medical reader of *Main Street* an appealing chapter is that describing an amputation. . . .") They had medicine in common. A lean redhead in his late thirties, Lewis came from a family of Minnesota doctors—father, grandfather, brother, uncle—and was fascinated by it perforce. He and Fishbein both liked to raise a glass, too, the difference being that the latter could handle it while the other too often could not. In any case, at about the same time he was shooting off provocative warnings to the California medical board about John Brinkley, Fishbein was also showing his new chum Lewis around town.

In the 1920s, Paris wasn't the only moveable feast. With Chicago in the throes of Art Deco fever, the stodgiest institutions acquired the romance of nightclubs, and as for the real thing—places like the Trianon, billed as "America's most luxurious ballroom"—anyone who forgot his hip flask could get drunk on the decor. Fishbein's particular passion was the theater, dating back to his student days when he earned extra money toting Sarah Bernhardt on- and offstage, and he was always taking visitors to play and movie palaces, where the spectacular houses themselves were half the show. He loved cards, too, including poker games at Ben Hecht's North Side apartment with Sandburg and Clarence Darrow.

Through Fishbein, Lewis got a taste of all these amusements, plus something more: an introduction to the gang at Schlogl's.

Set on the North Side under the clatter of an elevated train, Schlogl's restaurant was a German stein-and-stag type of haunt with dark scrolled wood, gold leaf, cloudy mirrors, and ropes of cigar smoke. On the tables were butter in pound blocks and baskets of fresh rye; on the plates were the expected—Wiener schnitzel, apple pancakes—and the unexpected: eels in aspic, roast venison, and "owls to order." But the real hub of the action wasn't in the kitchen. It was in the back right corner of the dining area, where a raucous, big-shoulders version of the Algonquin Round Table regularly convened.

In those days Chicago could lay claim to the headiest literary scene in America, capable of battles, as H. L. Mencken put it, "full of tremendous whoops, cracks, wallops and deviltries, with critics pulling the nose at critics, and volunteers going over the top in swarms, and the air heavy with ink, ears, typewriters, adjectives, chair legs and strophes from the Greek Anthology." At Schlogl's this close-quarters combat had been going on since 1916 with a crowd that had grown to include Hecht, Sandburg, Sherwood Anderson (known for his soft voice and atrocious socks), Edgar Lee Masters, and a score of flaring rushlights, now forgotten, the boys from the local press with the quickest minds and the sharpest elbows. If they had ever been quarantined there all together, many would likely have died of conceit or insecurity, but the talk was exciting because it pushed beyond gossip; these men (it was all men) made a point of it. Topics discussed ranged from the metaphysical poets to the psychology of the Russians to the folkways of the Chippewa, with the ignorant or inebriated often advancing the strongest opinions. Men scribbled articles in the midst of the ruckus. Someone else might pull out a ukulele. As for Fishbein himself, Ben Hecht remembered him as a talker among talkers there, "a medical savant with a passion for oratory. His pale bald dome gleamed at our table like a beacon of knowledge. He was a man of many charms, high among them being his inability to win at any card game."

Lewis was loudly welcomed at Schlogl's, and thereafter at private parties thrown by members of the crew. Drunk, he told wonderful stories about when he'd been drunk before. He improvised playlets in which he acted all the parts, and he made the ladies scream by going out high apartment windows and creeping along the ledge.

As they got to know each other better, Lewis and Fishbein didn't always see eye to eye. The novelist told the doctor he'd go further if he changed his name; *Fishbein* was too Jewish. Fishbein retorted that it was gentile prejudice that needed changing. Over lunch he once told

Lewis about the AMA's bulging quack files, urged him to look through them and write a book centered on medicine. The author declined.

His head was full of another subject—the very thing, in fact, that had brought him to Chicago. Lewis had come to visit the nation's leading champion of the labor movement, Eugene V. Debs, because he planned to base the hero of his next novel on him. A provocateur of great courage, Debs had been a five-time presidential candidate on the Socialist Party ticket, last running in 1920 from an Atlanta prison, where he had been jailed for agitating against the war. His unique campaign—"For President, Convict No. 9653"—had earned him almost a million votes. But after a lifetime of political struggle and two years of prison, he was physically and emotionally spent. He was recovering now, or trying to, at the Lindlahr Sanitarium in suburban Chicago, a place recommended to him by a disciple of Dr. Albert Abrams, the great rheostat dynamizer quack.

Fishbein regarded Abrams as "the world's second greatest charlatan," after Brinkley, and he held Henry Lindlahr—head of the sanitarium to which Debs had repaired—in almost equal contempt. This was due in part to Lindlahr's use of Abrams's oscilloclast as part of the treatment program, but the sanitarium was chiefly famous for its "naturopathy" regimen, which Fishbein detested just as much. Once mildly fashionable, by the early 1920s naturopathy barely clung to life with about a dozen schools nationwide. The coursework (which Fishbein enjoyed reciting) included sysmotherapy, gluckokinesis, zone therapy, physicultopathy, astrological diagnosis, practical sphincterology, phrenological physicology, spectrochrome therapy, iridiagnosis, tension therapy, and naprapathy. In short, naturopathy was a sort of elephant's graveyard or jumble sale of all things quackish—embracing, as the editor put it, "every form of healing that offers opportunity for exploitation." As for Dr. Lindlahr himself, the naturopath-chiropractor was a graduate of the notorious National Medical University of Chicago, which Fishbein classed as "a low-grade institution, virtually a diploma mill" and a local health official once called "the worst place in the city."

How, then, could a man of Debs's stature be sucked in? Dr. Fishbein believed that mavericks like Debs—trailblazers, people who think for themselves—were often unusually susceptible to quackery because they tended to carry their independent thinking outside their areas of expertise. ("The freethinker in politics is likely to fall for freethinking science just as he falls for political panaceas.") The editor conveyed the substance of these views to Lewis and urged him in the strongest terms, whatever course he pursued with his novel, to persuade Debs to flee the sanitarium.

Unconvinced, Lewis went out there to see for himself.

On a slow day at Schlogl's, Carl Sandburg came in, ordered a ham on rye, and settled at the big table with a few fellow loiterers. A reporter for the *Daily News,* Sandburg was an unusual type among the Schlogl's gang, and respected for it: he wasn't jazzy or up-to-date, but slower spoken, more like a plowman with a Ph.D. After a few bites of his sandwich, he took some pages out of his pocket.

"I've been writing some stories for the kids at home," he said, "reading to them at night and this is as far as I've got. I'll read it to you." And he did, a story about a little boy who lived in the Village of Liver and Onions.

There were others as well, with titles like "Three Boys With Kegs of Molasses and Secret Ambitions" and "How to Tell Corn Fairies If You See Them."

"Are you going to publish them?" somebody asked.

"I hadn't thought of that. I've just been writing them for the children."

But that wasn't true. Sandburg had secret ambitions of his own. Back home in his study, he wrote to his publisher, Alfred Harcourt, discussing window displays and trying to figure out how to pitch the publicity for this new collection, called *Rootabaga Stories.*

"Do we want some reviewer to say, 'This book is better than goat glands'?"

12

L ike a doormat lover, Milford took him back again.

In the fall of 1922 Brinkley was back at the old stand, in the afterglow of a second embarrassment. Dissecting his state license application, the California medical board had found his résumé riddled with lies and discrepancies. He had not graduated from Bennett Medical College, as he claimed. There was no record of his ever having attended Milton Academy in Baltimore. The list went on. Relying perhaps on the powerful friendship of Harry Chandler—and given the thousands of other quacks who thrived there unmolested—Brinkley had had every reason to think that the licensing board would apply its usual sleepy standards to him. Instead he had been vetted with microscopic diligence. That most of this diligence originated with Morris Fishbein, who had fed his findings to the board, Brinkley was still unaware. He did know or sense, however, that the AMA was mixed up in it somehow, and he viewed that organization henceforth with a settled loathing.

Gone from California, he was hardly forgotten. Dr. Leo Stanley at San Quentin had shifted to goat-gland tests of his own, work that was tracked and applauded by the *Los Angeles Times*—"Criminality Is Cured." To these efforts Brinkley did not object. What infuriated him were the fly-by-night clinics that sprang up in L.A. the moment he left, their proprietors claiming to have learned the mysteries of goat-gland grafting from the master himself. Brinkley had to publish a large, indignant advertisement denouncing them as quacks.

But . . . spilt milk, ever onward. To Minnie he said, "The harder they hit me, the higher I bounce." He never sulked long when there was money to be made. And these days there was plenty out there.

Raccoon coats might be all the rage, and flappers and saucy slang ("None of your beeswax!"), but America had not forgotten what made it great. When a Baltimore boy named Avon Foreman set a record sitting atop a flagpole, the mayor praised him in terms of traditional values: "The grit and stamina evidenced by your endurance from July 20th to 30th, a period of 10 days, 10 hours, 10 minutes and 10 seconds atop of the 22 foot pole in the rear of your home shows that the old pioneer spirit of early America is being kept alive by the youth of today." More important, the chasing of wealth—perhaps the nation's most traditional value of all—was more frenetic than ever. "Materialism flourished like an evangelical cult," as one historian put it, and not just among tycoons: depending on his line of work, the average American's paycheck rose 20 to 50 percent between 1915 and 1925, opening up new vistas in getting and spending, and triggering in turn many devious schemes for taking that money away. Brinkley was as much a creature of his times as he was a predator upon them. What set him apart was his resilience and brilliance.

It was as if California had never been. That fall he mailed out thousands of flyers explaining how Milford was the perfect location for his work, the "ideal combination: modernity set in the midst of truly rural peace and quiet." Minnie pointed out to reporters that all the most fashionable sanitariums in England were located in the countryside—reinforcing which, Brinkley added a coat of arms to his stationery, with a knight, shield, flowers, and vines in vivid gold and eggplant. A newspaper photo of the time shows him romping with his English water spaniel.

He expanded the hospital. The new lobby had chairs and couches, figured carpet, chandeliers, and wide windows with drapes tied back to let the sunshine in. New ads for the place were grandly redundant: "It is modern throughout, private rooms with bath, and the latest and most modern equipment, telephone in every room, private rooms, reading rooms, lounging rooms, large spacious lobby and dining room, modern drug store and barber shop . . ."

His torrential pamphleteering overwhelmed any bad publicity from the West Coast. It did more than tout the hospital; it tunneled into the psyche. In this form letter—dated October 25, 1922—he asks the recipient to send him ten cents for a copy of *Rejuvenation* magazine:

> My Dear Friend:
>
> If you agree that you and myself were created by Omnipotence for a purpose on [*sic*] this universe and that our existence here is not a happenstance, then it is our duty singly and collectively to leave this World a better place than we found it. . . . I believe my surgical work is fifty years ahead of the times when it comes to curing insanity, diseases of old age, assisting bright minds and valuable men and women to remain here and finish work of value to the coming generation. . . .
>
> I have selected you to assist in a small way. I have selected you as one of God's creatures to help spread this message of Hope to a suffering World, and this is your opportunity to, in a small way, do your share. When you have read the magazine kindly pass it to others that they may be informed of its message of Truth and Hope. Please do this now while it is fresh in your mind and before you forget it.

This was just one letter in a purposed series—no need to mention business yet.

Meanwhile, his staff busily gathered and published testimonials. There was nothing innovative about this strategy. Testimonials had always been the alpha and omega of nonestablished medicine, to the vast annoyance of its foes. Arthur Cramp created a poster—TESTIMONIALS ARE WORTHLESS—for national distribution. Fishbein ran a recurring feature in *JAMA,* a two-page spread: on one side, a reproduction of the testimonial, with a picture of who gave it and the disease they were miraculously cured of; on the facing page, that same person's death certificate, cause of death, same disease. But it was almost impossible to make any headway with the public on this front. "When the average American sets out to buy a horse or a box of cigars, he is a model of caution," wrote Samuel Hopkins Adams, but when seeking health, "the most precious of all possessions," the shopper seemed to lose his mind. "An admiral whose puerile vanity has betrayed him into a testimonial; an obliging and conscienceless senator; a grateful idiot in some remote hamlet; a renegade doctor or a silly woman who gets a bonus of a dozen photographs for her letter—any of these are sufficient to lure the hopeful patient to his purchase. He wouldn't buy a second-hand bicycle on the affidavit of any of them, but he will give up his dollar and take his chance of poison on a mere newspaper statement which he doesn't even investigate." Add to that the fact that 80 percent of all physical afflictions, if not actively interfered with, heal themselves; add to that the placebo effect; and any half-bright quack could thrive for years.

The most majestic testimonial Brinkley scored that fall of 1922 came from U.S. Senator Wesley Staley of Colorado. He acclaimed Dr. and Mrs. Brinkley "two of the finest people and the greatest benefactors to mankind on earth. . . . I wear goat glands and am proud of it." Eventually the doctor collected more than a hundred such tributes into a book, *Shadows and Sunshine*—before-and-after letters from grateful goat-gland patients, male and female.

But he couldn't rest there. The game was too crowded. "In the last two years," the *New York Times* observed, "the reading public has become pretty well accustomed to the almost continuous hysterical manifestation of concern for its glandular welfare. A war-ridden world has given place to a gland-ridden world." Every time you turned around someone else was getting "Steinached" or "Voronized," while the debate raged over which, if either, of them worked. That very summer, while Brinkley was in California, yet another rejuvenation doctor had grabbed headlines in Chicago, vexing the Milford Messiah no end.

Why Chicago again? Two reasons: first, the doctor in question was a leading disciple of Dr. Frank Lydston, who worked there; second, Chicago was also the home of Harold F. McCormick, multimillionaire heir to the International Harvester fortune and husband of Edith Rockefeller, daughter of John D. In a peccadillo that Orson Welles would later filch for *Citizen Kane,* the fifty-one-year-old McCormick had fallen in love with "nonsinging diva" Ganna Walska of Poland. Walska wasn't the dewy sort; she had already been married several times and was proud of it. (According to one then-current story, Walska had boasted, "Every man proposes to me the second he meets me," to which another lady rejoined, "Yes, but what does he propose?") Nevertheless, McCormick was besotted, and in 1920 he had used his position on the Chicago Opera Company board to ram her into the leading role in *Zaza.* He then hired a world-class voice coach to make it work. It didn't. Crowned "one of the biggest disasters of 1920," *Zaza* sent Walska fleeing back to Europe with McCormick right behind her. Two years later he was still her poodle. Having him get a gland transplant was apparently her idea, although one paper attributed it to a chance encounter with a European specialist:

"[McCormick] explained to the scientist that he was trying to keep young by a rigid regime of diet and exercise. The exercise included outdoor sports and gymnastic work in which he became so expert that he could turn fifteen handsprings in succession. The scientist told him . . . that such violent exercise was too strenuous for a man of more than forty, and advised him to study the subject of gland transplantation."

To perform the operation, the magnate settled on Dr. Victor Lespinasse, a Chicago urologist who had studied with Lydston. McCormick tried to keep the whole thing quiet—unsuccessfully.

SECRET OPERATION ON H. F. M'CORMICK
Family Refuses to Say Whether His Stay in Hospital
Is for Gland Transplanting
Keeping Young His Hobby
—*New York Times*, June 18, 1922, front page

The *Chicago Herald-Examiner* had also gotten wind of the story and put a squad of reporters on it. This was, after all, the city that gave birth to *The Front Page*—written by working reporters Ben Hecht and Charles MacArthur, it would hit Broadway four years later—and the newshounds who went after the McCormick story might as well have been auditioning for it. On a tip, they appeared en masse at the information desk of Wesley Memorial Hospital, where one of them falsely identified himself as Detective Sergeant Thomas A. Mullen and demanded to see the register. What they discovered led them to converge on Dr. Lespinasse's house after midnight, ringing the bell and throwing pebbles at his window to rouse him. When he finally raised the sash and discovered who they were, Lespinasse slammed it shut again and phoned his patient at once to warn him. But an *Examiner* man was already on a nearby pole, tapping into the doctor's line.

Still, details remained infuriatingly sketchy, with McCormick sealed off in a private wing at the hospital. Rumors flew. One had the patient receiving new testicles from an Illinois blacksmith, which gave rise to this barroom ditty:

> Under the spreading chestnut tree,
> The village smithy stands;
> The smith a gloomy man is he,
> McCormick has his glands.

Then came a report in the *New York Times*, apparently with harder information: ". . . it has been fairly well established that with Mr. McCormick in the same hospital there is an unidentified stranger, a virile youth of formidable stature and highly developed athletic propensities, carefully selected for his physical attainments. It is hinted around the hospital that the unidentified youth has acquired some of Mr. McCormick's wealth in return for a sacrifice on behalf of Mr. McCormick."

Two days later Lespinasse finally spoke to the press. He denied that he had given McCormick a human-gland operation. Few believed him. Aside from its being the doctor's stock-in-trade, why else would his patient be paying him fifty thousand dollars? But whatever the physician's motivation—discretion, petulance, guile—his denial was enough to ignite another wild round of crackpot speculation. ("Was it transplantation of some animal gland, such as a goat's or a monkey's, or was [it] some miraculous substance yet unknown to the medical world generally, but discovered by Dr. Lespinasse?")

Eventually McCormick slunk away without ever giving the facts.

The "miraculous substance" theory, however, got enough play to give an extra boost to the nonsurgical gland industry, which by 1922 was going great guns. Essentially this was a revival of the Brown-Sequard approach from thirty years before, old wine in new bottles, but it had enormous appeal for those too poor or too apprehensive for a full laying on of glands. Brinkley had this angle covered already with his Special Gland Emulsion, which he sold mail-order for a hundred dollars, rectal syringe included. But again, look at the competition! It started with variations on his own work, like the goat-gland suppositories for women being sold in San Francisco, and went from there: the Youth Gland Chemical Laboratories of Illinois ("Feeding Actual Gland Substance Direct to the Glands"), the Vital-O-Gland Company of Denver, Glandine, Glandex, Glandtone, Glandol . . .

Meanwhile, reports were emerging from France of simple replacement breakthroughs, which if true could eliminate the need for gland transplants altogether. There was Dr. Cruchet of Bordeaux, who claimed success rejuvenating patients by giving them blood transfusions from animals, news soon disputed by Dr. Jaworski of Paris, who claimed the same for his technique, injecting small amounts of a young person's blood into an older person. Jaworski's prize patient was octogenarian Armand Guillaumin, one of the last surviving Impressionist painters. Known for his extravagant use of color, like his friend Van Gogh, Guillaumin was now a grand old man of French art, so the eyes of the nation were upon him as he received injections of a maiden's blood in what was billed as a revolutionary "blood marriage." Some questioned how novel the treatment actually was—Pope Innocent VII in the fifteenth century had sought to revivify himself by drinking the blood of little boys—but Guillaumin's friends and family said it had done wonders for him.

How was Brinkley to rise above all this clamor he had helped so much to create? His brain, to quote a writer for *Collier's,* was "busier than an electric fan."

13

Late that same eventful summer of 1922, a stranger appeared in Fishbein's office with a letter of introduction from H. L. Mencken. He was Paul DeKruif, a Bunyanesque bacteriologist and science writer who had just quit his job at the Rockefeller Institute in New York. Prior to that, DeKruif (pronounced "de-krife") had fought under General Pershing against Pancho Villa, then worked in France during the Great War doing microbe studies on the effects of poison gas. People who met him were often struck by the size of his neck, which was thick as a post. Mencken once described him as "a natural enthusiast [who] embraced every new idea with roars."

Fishbein made an equal impression on DeKruif, as he recorded in his memoir, *The Sweeping Wind:* "Brilliant is the most frequent description of Dr. Fishbein today and brilliant was how he impressed me in 1922. Though not yet in his middle thirties and only an associate editor, his hand was firm at the controls of the *Journal of the American Medical Association. . . .* He held me in awe of him."

Too ornery for steady employment, DeKruif had come to Chicago to pursue a project of his own: an exposé of bogus medicines, those peddled not by quacks but by respected drug companies. He was a fraud buster intent on popularizing his findings—in other words, he was Fishbein's kind of man, so much so that the doctor was drawn into doing something mildly uncharacteristic. In the coming years Fishbein would be accused, occasionally with justice, of toeing the establishment line too blindly. This time, at least, he was willing to risk the displeasure of some *JAMA* advertisers, though he did it in a way that protected doctors themselves.

When DeKruif asked what Fishbein knew about dubious medicines from major companies, the editor launched into a monologue. DeKruif was surprised at the "fantastic precision" of his outpourings. "His narrative of the fooling of physicians by drugmongers was convincing, amusingly anecdotal, and, in its learning, encyclopedic. I felt as if caught in a didactic avalanche and then run over by a steamroller upon reaching the bottom. And yet, strangely, when this brilliant briefing was over, I remembered little of what Dr. Fishbein had said." DeKruif wasn't the only one over the years to find his new friend, at least on first acquaintance, more an experience than a source of facts.

After their session Fishbein took DeKruif down the hall to meet Dr. Cramp, introduced the two, and departed.

Cramp pulled bottles off his shelves, one after another, and set them in front of his visitor. DeKruif scanned labels and sniffed corks with mounting excitement. There was plenty here to expose, thanks to the declining force of the Pure Food and Drug Act. Since Prohibition, tonics had been taking in a lot of homeless alcohol. DeKruif peppered Cramp with questions.

While they were talking, Sinclair Lewis came up in the elevator.

For the past week or so Lewis had been making pilgrimages to the Lindlahr Sanitarium in Elmhurst to visit Eugene Debs. The great crusader was wan and gaunt, but his bony hands gripped Lewis's shoulders the first time they met. "Gene really is a Christ spirit," Lewis wrote his wife. "He is infinitely wise, kind, forgiving—yet the devil of a fighter." That first meeting lasted several hours. Lewis told him of his plan to write a novel about the labor movement (working title: *Neighbor*) with a hero modeled largely on the old socialist himself. Flattered, Debs told him some yarns from his past, like the time he led a strike against the Great Northern Railroad.

As for the sanitarium itself, Lewis found himself half-impressed, despite Fishbein's scorn for it. Again writing to his wife, Grace, the novelist described the regimen there: ". . . barefoot walking in the dewy grass at 6 A.M. (ooooooo)!—breakfast one plum, one apfel, & one pear and if you MUST be carnal, one tepid cup of Postum; supper (me—I et it, with Gene) spinach, Norske bread, milk, & watermelon. . . . But it is quiet there, & pleasant under the trees, & probably good for Debs." (Certainly good for him was the close proximity of Carl Sandburg, who by chance lived with his wife and daughters just three blocks away. Several times during his stay Debs slipped away to visit him, and the two men, who fit together like a pair of old shoes, strolled under the elms on Sandburg's property having a proletarian chin-wag.)

But then Lewis began having doubts. First about his project: perhaps he didn't want to write a labor novel after all. He had been attending some Chicago union meetings as research, and the more laborites he talked to, the more they bored him. The caustic bard of *Main Street* and *Babbitt* found too many of Debs's sainted workingmen "plain boobs."

Moreover, thanks to the relentless Fishbein, Lewis's confidence in the sanitarium was slipping, too, and with it some of his respect for Debs. To Grace, August 26: "[T]he kind of credulity which permits a Debs to fall for a Lindlahr system with its hysteric food, its chiropractic, its phony 'electronic' treatments (you should hear Dr. Fishbein on the subject!) is shocking to me. However irrational I may be at times, I worship rationality more than I do faith."

Such was Lewis's state of mind when he arrived at Fishbein's office late in the afternoon. The editor, who had some of the instincts of a Washington hostess, took him by the elbow and bore him down the hall to meet the newcomer. As DeKruif recalled it: "Here now in the door of Dr. Cramp's office there loomed, in tow of Dr. Fishbein, a young redheaded man, very tall and slightly stooped, nervous, his face spotty red as if about to explode into a dermatosis. His light blue eyes fixed sharply on me for a moment, then peered, dartingly, round the office."

While Fishbein did the introductions, Lewis's eyes roamed the rows of exotic tonics on display. He began to explore. "Off the shelf came a bottle," DeKruif recalled, "twitching in Mr. Lewis's nervous hands. It was a big vial of bitters made in Baltimore. Sinclair Lewis peered at the bottle's label.

"My God, it's high in alcohol," he exclaimed. "Do you mean they let people buy that over the counter in drugstores?" Then he whirled round and fixed me with his fierce blue eyes.

"You're an investigator, you're a scientist, do you dare to taste this bottle's contents?" asked Lewis.

"Do I dare to *taste* it?" I answered. "I'll drink all of it!" No, no, he wasn't asking me to be that foolish; but as Dr. Fishbein moved to intercept it the bottle was at my mouth and, head thrown back, with gusto and bravado I gulped all the bitter-tasting stuff with one mighty swig, choking and coughing at the end of it. There was a look of real concern on the faces of Drs. Cramp and Fishbein and a look of alarm—tinged with admiration—on the spotty visage of the great author.

Fishbein remembered it differently. He said DeKruif had been in Cramp's office sampling bottles all afternoon. Either way, the result was the same. When the editor took both men home to his Michigan Avenue apartment for dinner, DeKruif began the evening in prayer position at the toilet. After a short nap he awoke refreshed.

Over dinner the three men talked, apropos of DeKruif's last job in New York, about medical research—what a difficult field it was, hamstrung by politics, jealousies, and low pay. No wonder so many topflight men abandoned it for private practice.

The wine flowed.

Whether prompted by guilt, a need for fresh air, or just the mysterious logic of an alcoholic, Lewis suddenly insisted that they all go visit Debs. The others tried to talk him out of it. It was after dark. It was too far. He wouldn't listen. Moments later, DeKruif wrote, they were heading out the door, "propelled by Red, who was volcanic."

Being wedged all three in the back of a cab proved insanely irritating. According to a Lewis biographer, "At the intersection of Van

Buren, Ashland, and Jackson streets, [Lewis and DeKruif] got out of the cab and broke into a tussle, the huge, burly man and the long, thin one, and Lewis, shoved against the cab, managed both to tear his trousers and to cut his leg. Fishbein knew the pharmacist in a drugstore on that corner, and they went in there, attended to the leg, and continued."

There was a sudden rainstorm, and their taxi hit another car. When they finally arrived at the sanitarium it was after midnight. The building had a wide wraparound porch clustered about with shrubbery, and there they sat with Debs, who supplied the whiskey (he wasn't the perfect patient after all) while the eaves dripped and the four men talked deep into the night. Fishbein inveighed against quackery in general and naturopathy in particular; against humbugs in general and Dr. Lindlahr in particular; and Lewis, now in complete accord, added his voice, urging Debs to leave. All in vain. His response was a radiant declaration of faith in Lindlahr and all he stood for.

The visitors left around 4 A.M. On the ride home, with Debs's folly fresh in mind, Fishbein seized the chance. He again pressed Lewis to dump his idea of a labor novel and write about a hero doctor instead. Or a medical researcher maybe, one of those men they were talking about at dinner, in lone pursuit of scientific truth. DeKruif backed the idea, and finally Lewis agreed. He asked Fishbein to collaborate as technical adviser. Whether the overworked editor chose to decline (as he claimed), or Lewis gracelessly yanked the offer later and asked DeKruif instead (as he claimed), the novelist and the unemployed scientist became a team. In the weeks that followed they settled on a bacteriologist hero and a tropical locale, and set off together to the West Indies on a research tour. Mencken wrote Fishbein from New York that he had "poured them on the boat."

What emerged from it all was *Arrowsmith*, winner of the 1926 Pulitzer Prize.

14

How would Brinkley crush his rivals? He probably knew already. The moment he'd seen Harry Chandler's radio station, the doctor was hooked. Getting a broadcasting license, one of the first in the Midwest, was a snap in those days, and he broke ground on his studio and tower in early 1923.

Through a glass darkly he saw an empire.

Few others had such foresight. To most Americans then, radio was like fire after its discovery by cavemen: it was fabulous, astounding . . . now what? Since the first valiant broadcast of the 1920 presidential election returns by KDKA in Pittsburgh, great things had been predicted for this new medium: that it would cure the deaf, that it would bring world peace. But as 1922 drew to a close, the roughly six hundred licensed stations in America were still mere fireflies; for the listener with his clunky headphones, just picking up scraps of a saxophone solo from who knew where was a thrill. And the fundamental questions remained unanswered: What sort of broadcasting did the public want? Who should give it to them? And who was going to pay for it?

By mid-1923 an inchoate demand for good programming (whatever that might mean) was rising fast, partly in reaction to the loonies and professional attention-attracters flooding into the breach. A certain W. K. "Hello World" Henderson had started a station in Shreveport, Louisiana, to deliver profanity-strewn rants for "the greater glory of God and the damnation of chain stores." Someone calling himself the Great DeWese parachuted from a plane with a microphone so he could describe his sensations on the way down. An Illinois preacher informed his radio flock that the earth was flat, having just taken a boat ride around the world and seen "no evidence of curving."

In short, radio was begging for help. It needed big ideas. And over the next fifteen to twenty years, Dr. Brinkley would have some of the biggest.

Like any great commander, he could spot and channel talent—in this case, people in other fields who cared nothing for goat glands but couldn't resist a professional challenge. One of these he hired as chief engineer: James O. Weldon of Dallas, Texas. Weldon, who could have passed for Fred Astaire's brother, was a near genius in this fledgling technology. During the summer of 1923 he designed and built transmitters from scratch, installed them in a small brick building just outside Milford, and oversaw construction of two three-hundred-foot towers nearby. He was so good at his job that with station KFKB ("Kansas First, Kansas Best") still months from completion, the Brinkleys put the whole thing in his hands, boarded an ocean liner, and embarked on a goat-gland demonstration tour of Asia.

Their first stop was China, where Dr. Brinkley performed the operation on the president of the Bank of Peking, among others— four men and one woman, as Minnie remembered it, including "the uncle of the boy who would have been the emperor had the country not gone republic." It was here the *Chinese Press* hailed their new visitor as "the Burbank of Humanity." After that, journeying south with Minnie, the doctor bought some stolen antiques, inspected a colony of eunuchs in Saigon, and circumcised the Prince of Siam on a ship in the Malacca Strait.

While they were thus engaged, a new book back in the States was causing quite a stir: *Crystallizing Public Opinion* by Edward L. Bernays. Billed as an operating manual for a new profession the author called "public relations," it dovetailed almost exactly with Brinkley's own evolving vision.

Bernays wasn't the first man ever to buff an image; a decade earlier, Ivy Lee had oil baron John D. Rockefeller passing out dimes to poor children in hopes of countering the common view that he was a heartless bastard. But where Lee saw himself as a short-term fixer, Bernays saw down the centuries. A short braggart with a tremendous mustache, he would come to be known as the father of spin.

In his 1923 book and its follow-up, *Propaganda,* Bernays put forth the arresting notion that public relations could serve as a replacement for God. Staggered by the slaughter in the recent world war, he said, millions had fallen away from religion. Groping in an existential fog, they craved direction, a sense of purpose. Who could supply it? Why, big business. In an era when, thanks to advances in the study of human psychology, "it is now possible to control and regiment the masses according to our will without their knowing it," America's corporations had not only the opportunity but the duty to wield this power. Without "publicity as an instrument of control," a godless world would dissolve in chaos.

PR as a moral imperative: to the average captain of industry, could any idea be more appealing? Suddenly Bernays was a star of the social sciences—quite on a par in some circles with his uncle, Sigmund Freud, whose name he dropped with regularity. They were two sides of the same coin, Bernays liked to say, and the press helped him. "The great Viennese doctor," the *Atlantic Monthly* explained, "is interested in releasing the pent-up libido of the individual; his American nephew is engaged in releasing (and directing) the suppressed desires of the crowd."

But one man out there didn't need fancy lessons in "the engineering of consent." Before he left for Asia, Brinkley already had in place at least four men in four different towns—Milford, Topeka, Chicago, and New York—whose sole and specific job it was to exalt him in the eyes of the world. Smart, resourceful, they suggested angles and even supplied stories to newspapers, reports of fictional events both at home and overseas. Awed Americans ceased chewing their morning toast as they read that His Highness, the Maharajah Thakou Galub of Morvi, would be traveling to Milford from distant India to receive his goat glands. On April 21, 1923, the following appeared in the Gettysburg *Star and Sentinel:*

Gland Transplantation Now Used by Japan to Put Aged Infirm Back at Work! High Class Goat Prices Soar

"Goat gland transplantation," the article began, "has been made compulsory in Japan by the government in order to rejuvenate aged charity patients. . . . Within the past few months more than 2,000 of these inmates have undergone the operation and are again earning their own living." Most had regained their eyesight and hair, ran the report, and Dr. W. H. Ballou of New York City ("a thoroughly informed scientist, to whom far things are near and strange things familiar") expatiated on Brinkley's eminence and skill. Of all the doctor's press agents, Ballou was the most sonorous and convincing. "The children of parents who have been endowed with goat glands," he once said, "are healthy and alert to an unusual degree. . . . New glands mean not only new vitality to men and women now living . . . but they actually mean better babies. I say that in this—in making possible a superior type of human being—Dr. Brinkley has made a discovery of the first importance to mankind."

Returning north through China, the doctor kept close tabs on the progress of his radio station through reports from Weldon and others. There was one snag after another since the local builders weren't entirely sure what a radio station was. Then a fire destroyed the site and they had to start over. Brinkley was unfazed. He spent hours in hotel rooms and aboard ship jotting down thoughts and doodling designs, then shooting them off to Weldon.

In Shanghai the Brinkleys boarded a French liner bound for Hong Kong. Before it cast off, city officials presented a fireworks display in honor of another passenger, Sir Robert Hotung, a British philanthropist who had helped fund the revolution against the old emperor. The dull booms of the rockets lasted well into the night, long after the ship had embarked. Sir Robert retired to his cabin, but Brinkley remained at the stern, gazing at the riot in the sky. Rapt, he stood alone at the rail until the last rocket was shot.

15

It was the strangest thing. Evelyn Lyons was lying in her own bed at home, recovering from minor injuries suffered in a car crash, when Dr. H. J. Hefnet tried to take her temperature. According to the hometown paper, the *Escanaba (Michigan) Daily Press,* "the mercury rose almost instantly to the top of the tube, and snapped the glass at the neck of the bulb." Nonplussed, her physician obtained another, sturdier thermometer from the U.S. Weather Bureau. He tried again. Her temperature read an astounding 118 degrees. Day after day the fever raged, never sinking below 114, yet the young woman remained unaccountably alive. Before long what began as a bit of queer gossip had claimed front pages across the nation. Other doctors who were called in confirmed the findings but could not explain them either. "Despite her condition she continues rational," Dr. Hefnet reported.

That was in early March 1923. For two weeks the patient's temperature averaged 115 degrees, by which time the town was up to its neck in reporters, quacks, astrologers, and health-food crazies of every stripe. Mailmen staggered in with sackloads of advice. The editor of a foreign-language newspaper promised Miss Lyons would be restored to health if she chewed an herb "known only to Syrians." A California woman revealed that the fever was being broadcast from Russia by "radio demons." Interestingly, it was mostly quacks who thought she was faking. The young lady received a number of letters, written as one con artist to another, offering to split the take if she would allow them to come and "heal" her. Meanwhile U.S. medical authorities consulted with European experts as the moist patient, prostrate in bed, received a stream of well-wishers. "I am tired, so tired of being sick," she told a visitor. "I'll be better soon, I know. But everyone has been so kind and thoughtful"—with a nod toward the encroaching jungle of bouquets and get-well cards—"that it is easy to be cheerful."

By the next gathering of the clan at Schlogl's, the "Hot Girl of Escanaba" was reportedly throwing herself in snowbanks to cool off. The editor of the *Chicago Daily News* asked Morris Fishbein, as their resident medical expert, what he thought. Fishbein said it was a hoax. His friends roared at him to prove it, and the newspaper offered to pay his way.

To reach Escanaba was a three-hundred-mile push due north along the shore of Lake Michigan. The rail line crawled through unbroken snow and pine forests, past Scandinavian settlements, mink, and eagles. After a two-day trip the train arrived in Escanaba and a man got off. He was short, plump, and implacable.

The town was entombed in snow. In the lobby of his hotel Fishbein found an elderly local toasting himself by the fire. Rubbing his chilled hands there, the doctor introduced himself and asked what townsfolk were saying about the famous fever. The old man told him the leading theory was "moonshine backfire."

Outside the Lyons house, a small crowd loitered dumbly in the cold. Fishbein's AMA credentials got him inside, where he was introduced to the patient's exhausted mother. Upstairs he met Evelyn herself, tragic in bed. Her coughing and flailing were worse now, broken by spells of unconsciousness.

He touched her forehead. It was as hot as a Mexican sidewalk. Breathing shallow, pulse quick. Fishbein asked Miss Lyons a few questions while he took readings from oral and rectal thermometers—and then resorted to the overwhelmingly obvious ploy of leaving the room, closing the door, and squatting down to peek through the keyhole, Restoration comedy–style. He had to watch so long his foot went to sleep, but at last he saw what he was waiting for.

Then he burst in, other doctors at his back, for the discovery scene.

Escanaba's "Fever Girl" Is Branded as World Champion "Hysterical Malingerer"

A flesh colored hot water bottle was the secret of a hoax, by which Miss Evelyn Lyons of Escanaba, Mich., had been able to convince doctors for three weeks that she had a temperature of 114 degrees or higher, although apparently in good health, it was asserted tonight by Dr. Morris Fishbein, associate editor of the *Journal of the American Medical Association,* who related the investigation he made of the case.

"The woman, who had once been a nurse, concealed a small hot-water bottle in her bed," he said, "and through pretended fits of coughing and hysteria, managed to place the thermometer on the bottle long enough to drive the mercury to the desired point, where it remains in medical thermometers until shaken down." Breaking in upon her, Dr. Fishbein said, "We demanded the hot-water bottle and she declared she was insulted, but after some trouble she brought [it] out. . . . With the exception of hysteria, there is nothing wrong with Miss Lyons."

Excuses were offered for the shamefaced doctors and everyone else she had duped for more than a fortnight. The water bag had been manipulated, one report said, "with all the cleverness and skill of a polished conjurer," helped along by "her histrionic ability . . . and a never-ending supply of cunning." Excuses were made for Miss Lyons: that she had been disappointed in an affair of the heart, that the car crash had perhaps bruised her brain. What the success of her ruse mostly revealed was mankind's hunger for any scrap of magic. The fact remained, everyone involved looked like a dunce except for Morris Fishbein.

Partly to cover its own embarrassment, the press puffed Dr. Fishbein as hard as they had once puffed Miss Lyons. One paper likened his feat to exploding Sir Frederick Cook's claim of discovering the North Pole. All in all, the hoax was one of the biggest news stories of 1923.

It was also the defining moment of Fishbein's career. Along with making him famous as a fraud buster extraordinaire, the case fixed him in a role he would revel in for years to come: the face, the popularizer, the lord high priest of the AMA. There had never been such a figure before, but for the next twenty-five years or more, to the average citizen Morris Fishbein *was* American medicine.

On his return to Chicago he solidified his role by launching *Hygeia,* a sort of *JAMA* for the general public. He started a PR department as well (just a beat or two behind Brinkley) and threw open his phone lines to reporters seeking lively quotes on all things medical. But his reigning passion then and always would be putting quacks out of business. From the Hot Girl of Escanaba, it was an easy step to exposing charlatans in his own profession. He had a "real genius" for it, one colleague said, taking down "reckless and dangerous frauds with a gleam of relish in his eye."

Henceforth quack busting would no longer be an insular struggle among physicians but a blood sport the whole family could enjoy.

16

On March 1, 1923—while Miss Lyons tossed on her bed of pain—young Harry Thompson graduated from Chicago's Progressive College of Chiropractic, Dr. Henry Lindlahr, president. The newly minted Dr. Thompson received his diploma by mail. Inscribed in Latin on heavy paper with a wax seal, it was impeccable in every detail save one: it came from a different school. This document proclaimed Thompson an alumnus of the Kansas City College of Medicine and Surgery, Dr. Date R. Alexander, president.

Just how and why the switch took place was part of what Harry Thompson, an undercover reporter for the *St. Louis Star,* explained in his exposé on diploma mills, which burst upon the public in the fall of 1923. When word of the explosive series reached Dr. Brinkley, still on his triumphal tour of the Far East, it rang an unhappy bell, the diploma at issue being identical to the one Dr. Alexander had signed for him in 1915. Identical, in fact, to scores issued over the years to soda jerks, hod carriers, vacuum-cleaner salesmen, and park-bench pigeon feeders, none of whom had ever set foot inside a medical school.

When Thompson's series hit newsstands, there were as many as twenty-five thousand practicing physicians in America whose training was purely on paper. Not all had relied on diploma mills. Some had prolonged the careers of dead doctors by buying their diplomas from widows and assuming those names. An interstate ring had been stealing and selling the answers to state medical exams for years. The bulk of the fraud, however, flowed from the Kansas City College of

Medicine and Surgery and a handful of other schools, all purveyors of fake degrees. Of their phantom alumni Brinkley was one of the most highly trained, but that didn't make his diploma any less bogus. Mrs. Brinkley had bought one just like it.

Spurred by Thompson's revelations, the *Kansas City Journal Post* opened its own investigation into Dr. Date R. Alexander, the diploma-mill king. It discovered among other things that thanks to his regular payoffs to the Connecticut Eclectic Board, his so-called graduates did not approach licensing exams in that state "with the fear and trembling generally supposed to possess the applicant." His most recent crop of students had partied so hard the night before the test that a Hartford hotel was demanding repayment for smashed furniture.

Alexander's response to his newfound notoriety was to confront a reporter on the street. "You accused me of selling diplomas for $200," he said. "That is a deadly insult. I never charged less than $500." Whatever strange pleasure he was taking in disgrace Brinkley did not share. One result of the scandal was the blanket rescinding of all 167 medical licenses approved by the Connecticut Eclectic Board, his among them. For the first time he found himself in headlines he didn't want.

In early 1924 he cut his trip short and hastened home to Milford. Approaching the town, he beheld for the first time an antenna—his antenna—shooting up a hundred feet into the cornflower blue sky. But otherwise it was hardly the start he had envisioned: instead of taking the microphone to proclaim the new age of goat glands, he had to lead with an almost frantic defense of his professional integrity. His first broadcasts were mostly spent flaying yellow journalists and the stooges of the AMA, that graveyard of original thinking and "monopoly against the public interest."

It got worse. On July 8, 1924, the Associated Press reported from San Francisco that a grand jury had handed up nineteen indictments against men in the ever-spreading scandal, some for conferring fake medical degrees, others for being "beneficiaries of such operations." Brinkley's name was on the second list. The most concrete evidence against him derived from his doomed application for a California license, lies that Fishbein had exposed. Agents from Sacramento traveled fifteen hundred miles to arrest the goat-gland king.

To the governor of Kansas, Jonathan M. Davis, they presented their warrant for extradition.

Davis handed it back and told them to go home.

Asked why he refused to surrender Brinkley, the governor was disarmingly frank. "We people in Kansas get fat on his medicine," he said. "We're going to keep him here so long as he lives."

Crowing in triumph, Brinkley told his radio audience that the campaign against him had been "persecution . . . no more justified than the persecution of Christ." He mocked the AMA for backing the extradition effort and wasting, he claimed, $150,000 in its effort to ruin him. The new venue of radio was proving its might: no matter how many articles Fishbein wrote for *JAMA*, no matter how many speeches he gave denouncing "artificial rejuvenation as advertised by Brinkley and other such quacks," the editor's audience was tiny by comparison. Meanwhile, the worldwide publicity Brinkley had stirred with his Asian tour was reaping its harvest. Men arrived for goat-gland surgery from all over the globe: Europe, Canada, Australia, South Africa, South America. As the danger receded, Brinkley nestled into the pleasures of running KFKB, "the Sunshine Station in the Heart of the Nation"—a tag line, he said, "suggested by a crippled child." In fact, the child was in her mid-thirties, but she did have the perfect limp. Brinkley went to Barnes, Kansas, where he presented Rose Sedlacek with a wristwatch at a bandstand ceremony and gave her a ride in a plane.

17

In the year 1715, a volume entitled *Charlataneria Eruditorum—The Charlatanry of the Learned*—was published in Leipzig to great acclaim. Written by German author Johann Burckardt Mencken, it was an exposé of savants, those spouters of gimcrack erudition and bogus science (university professors usually) who then infested Europe. The frontispiece of the book was a picture of a medical charlatan surrounded by his assistants: a come-hither female, an acrobatic clown, and a figure who looked like a genie holding up a bottle of tonic. The parallel to academia was unambiguous.

More than two centuries later, in August 1923, a descendant of that author sat hammering his Underwood in his office on West Forty-fifth Street in New York. He was a compact man with a large head, his hair parted slightly to the left of center, with an unlit cigar in his teeth. The office was new, his magazine was new—so new the first issue hadn't appeared yet—but the willfully hideous Turkey-red carpet and large brass spittoon were old familiars from his last job.

He typed with two stabbing forefingers and spaced with his right elbow, surprising in a skilled pianist: "It goes without saying that I hope to make frequent forays against the quacks. Will you ever have time to do some articles?"

H. L. Mencken and Morris Fishbein had corresponded lightly over the past few years, fan letters back and forth, one editor to another. They weren't yet firm friends, nor had they ever collaborated. But with the *American Mercury,* this monthly he had just started with drama critic George Jean Nathan, Mencken hoped to give the 1920s a swift kick in the pants. He had been impressed by Fishbein's star turn in Escanaba and saw him as an ideal contributor.

Quack busters to the core, they were nonetheless radically different men. Fishbein saw himself first and foremost as a guardian of the public. Mencken, a connoisseur of fraud and rascality, treated quacks as no more degraded than anybody else, only more enterprising; if exposing them meant giving aid and comfort to the "booboisie," that was regrettable but couldn't be helped. He liked to claim that quacks had their good points, since they helped eliminate "persons of congenitally defective reasoning powers" from the gene pool. In fact, he wrote Fishbein, "What the country principally needs is a great increase in the death-rate, especially South of the Potomac."

Beneath the misanthropic wisecracks, however, Mencken took the health of one person seriously indeed. His hypochondria dated back at least to August 1915, when he checked into Johns Hopkins Hospital complaining of "a persistent sensation in the tongue." By the early twenties his private file marked "illnesses" was full to bursting. George Jean Nathan claimed that in the torrent of letters he received from Mencken over the years, not one failed to mention some "hypothetical physical agony," a cavalcade—quoting the sufferer now—of hay fever, hemorrhoids, "severe lumbago," "left tonsil hole . . . filled with scar tissue and other muck," sour stomach, laryngitis, "a small pimple inside the nose (going away)," a "warty tumor on the ball of the foot," and so on. A profound skepticism combined with a compulsion to wash his hands fifteen to twenty times a day gave Mencken a raging ambivalence toward the medical profession. One day it was all knaves and bandits; the next, as his brother August said, his attitude was "roughly parallel to a Catholic's attitude toward priests. . . . If a doctor told him to jump off a roof, he would have jumped." In the coming years, nothing would reveal that inner conflict more than the great battlefield of glands.

Fishbein was delighted at the prospect of sidelining for the *Mercury*. An amateur etymologist himself, he also volunteered to track down the roots of medical words for Mencken's ongoing masterwork on American language. (His first offering: "Dear Mr. Mencken, We are sending, under separate cover . . . our answer on the word 'moron.'")

Fishbein was hard at work on his first feature for the magazine, denouncing osteopathy as a quack cult, when the inaugural issue of the *Mercury* appeared in January 1924. One of its articles was entitled "The Pother About Glands" by pharmacologist and chemist L. M. Hussey, a sure sign there was still pother aplenty.

Sparked by the "senile-erotic" investigations of Dr. Charles Edouard Brown-Sequard, the renegade ex-Harvard professor who had rocked Paris with his testicular emulsion back in 1889, some legitimate breakthroughs in glandular research had occurred in the years since. The most spectacular came in 1921, when a pair of Canadian scientists isolated insulin, a hormone secreted in the pancreatic gland. This watershed in the treatment of diabetes netted Frederick Grant Banting and John James Richard Macleod a 1923 Nobel Prize. But the very magnificence of that achievement—see what glands can do!—added false fuel to the rejuvenation craze, and debunkers like Fishbein were more than ever outshouted and outgunned. Were all the boosters true believers? Not necessarily. An American doctor remarked that some of his colleagues were chiefly interested in rejuvenating their wallets. Still, breathless reports kept coming in—from Lille, France, for instance, claiming success with the "grafting of thyroid glands of criminals on backward children." Dr. William J. A. Bailey, director of the American Endocrine Laboratories, addressed a convention in New York as if he were being lifted into a spaceship. "We have cornered aberration, disease, old age, and in fact life and death themselves, in the endocrines!" he cried. With the right glandular tweak, Harry Thaw, the notorious killer of architect Stanford White, could be transformed from mental patient "into a useful citizen." Conversely, detectives would soon be using gland analysis to track down criminals, a technique already turning up in mystery stories like this one by Mignon Eberhart:

"What is it you—think you know about—this murderer?" asked Jenny.

"Why," said Tom, "we know several things quite definitely. . . . A touch of thymus, because there's a completely feelingless cruelty about Myrtle Shultz' murder. More than a little pituitary; for there's an extremity of cunning and daring. I expect," said Tom, "that some writing will crop up somewhere."

"Writing?"

"It's—among other things—the writing gland. When violently disordered, writing usually comes out in great quantities."

But if Joycean prose had a future, other forms might not. At a literary symposium in Manhattan, fear was expressed that the recapturing of youth and longer life spans could spell the end of introspective poetry, especially the sonnet. (What would the next Keats have to write about?)

Such was the climate when Hussey's article appeared in the *American Mercury*. A semiskilled mix of technical jargon and sarcasm, the report derided all methods of glandular rejuvenation, but particularly that of Dr. Steinach, who was then being bruited as a candidate for a Nobel Prize. "Has the *elixir vitae* been found at last?" A look at the facts "shatter[s] that theory completely."

Left unaddressed by Hussey, however, and by nearly every commentator of the day, was what this mad pounding after youth suggested about the snakier, more subterranean aspects of human nature. Such theorizing would have seemed tailor-made for the age of Freud, but the founder of psychoanalysis was keeping silent on the subject for reasons that emerged only after his death. Jung probed the link between glands and the "physiological structure of the brain," toyed with the notion of thoughts as "secretions of the brain," but his interest was more clinical than psychological. Even the daily press, set against the standards of our own day, was amazingly indifferent to just who these people flocking in for surgery were and what their motivations might be. Only those patients who insisted on making themselves conspicuous, like J. J. Tobias, even got their names in the paper.

Instead, rejuvenation rested on assumptions mushier than platitudes. The lure of youth? Life was happiness, so more life was more happiness: this was the level of public discourse. Anxieties up to and including terror of the grave simply weren't mentioned. But even exuberant souls like Tobias have their secrets. We don't need psychologists to tell us (though they do) that it is not only, or even primarily, happy people who are most eager to keep living. Those who experience life as grim and frightening often view death as even grimmer and more frightening. This is not to say that a hunger to stay alive is perverse, but merely that complexity and paradox rarely figure in popular delusions and the madness of crowds.

Similarly, for all the mass psychology theories emanating from Edward Bernays and others in the 1920s, no one seems to have framed the rejuvenation craze in those terms, as a cooperative fantasy. Yet a century and a half earlier the great Samuel Johnson had anatomized this dynamic perfectly: "[W]e go with expectation and desire of being pleased; we meet others who are brought by the same motives; no one will be the first to own the disappointment; one face reflects the smile of another, till each believes the rest delighted, and endeavours to catch and transmit the circulating rapture. In time, all are deceived by the cheat to which all contribute. The fiction of happiness is propagated by every tongue, and confirmed by every look, till at last all profess the joy which they do not feel, [and] consent to yield to the general delusion."

Thus the gabble over glands went on, and with every word John Brinkley became, to his radio listeners at least, that much more respectable.

Fishbein's byline appeared in the *Mercury*'s second issue, along with those of Eugene O'Neill, James M. Cain, and fellow Schlogl's carouser Sherwood Anderson. A cannonade against osteopathy, Fishbein's article had its merits even though, as with chiropractic, he was always better at reciting its disasters than tracking its advances. Mencken had just one measure of success—did the article make the target squeal like a stuck pig?—and that the piece accomplished. Guerrilla strikes like these would soon make the *Mercury* the "hip flask for the American mind," the defining magazine of the decade, for the war and its aftermath had made disillusionment (except over glands) fashionable even among the silly set. "Every flapper carries one of the green-backed journals conspicuously," one newspaper noted. ". . . To be surprised carrying the *American Mercury* or caught reading it at odd moments is now absolutely The Thing."

Fishbein fashionable—who would have predicted that? But like any great warrior, he was also making enemies wholesale, and they started to bite back. In June 1924, *Pearson's Magazine* blasted him as a sort of Machiavellian stooge. It accused him of finding quackery in "every method of healing except that of the school which has purchased the crafty pen of Morris Fishbein"—in other words, the AMA, that blind purveyor of surgery and pills with a membership to protect. At the same time, he diverted "public attention away from [the AMA's] own dungheap." The motive was simple: money.

The charges weren't entirely false. Like Toad of Toad Hall, Fishbein was prone to go overboard, and during his long career battling apostates and renegades, he tossed out the baby with the bathwater more than once. But the *Pearson's* article erred in claiming he did it for money. Others in the AMA might dream of economic monopoly, but Fishbein waged his holy war on alternative medicine largely for two reasons: to protect the public health and *pour le sport*. He called the AMA's quack-busting Bureau of Investigation "our fun department." For better and worse, he was congenitally intemperate.

Much like his new chum at the *Mercury*. Cementing their partnership, the Sage of Baltimore sent Fishbein a signed photo, which he hung on his office wall:

"To the philological pathologist, Morris Fishbein, from the pathological philologian, H. L. Mencken."

18

He was one of the great soloists of the Jazz Age. Each day Brinkley would sit at a small table with his gold-finished microphone, a grandfather clock ticking gravely behind him, and free-associate for hours in a mysterious soothsayer's voice that coasted across America's prairies and beyond. In the evenings whole families sat hunched toward their radios, like Moses listening to the burning bush: "Don't let your doctor two-dollar you to death. . . . Come to Dr. Brinkley. . . . Take advantage of our Compound Operation. . . . I can cure you the same as I did Ezra Hopkins of Possum Point, Missouri."

On he went, conjuring the great unseen to drop their dishrags, their tools, their nearest and dearest, and get to Milford on the double. The unadorned delivery made it hard to tell at first, but for sheer tactical variety his approach rivaled Cyrano's. He warbled ("A redbird and his mate are building their nest just outside my bedroom window. . . . Will you, for your health's sake, be with us this May?"). He scarified ("Many untimely graves have been filled with people who put off until tomorrow *what they should have done today*"). He used big words ("Watch your prostate for signs of hypertrophy and for a fibrous and sclerotic condition. If there is constipation, is there not also obstipation?"). He shamed ("Note the difference between the stallion and the gelding. The former stands erect, neck arched, mane flowing, chomping the bit, stamping the ground, seeking the female, while the gelding stands around half-asleep, cowardly, listless. . . . Men, don't let this happen to you").

He tried nearly everything, but he was smart enough not to over-reach. Brinkley rarely made the kinds of claims coming out of Europe, that glands would turn crones into debutantes or keep a man alive for centuries. His core audience was weather-hardened prairie folk. They weren't born yesterday. He kept the focus on sex.

As a consequence Doc Brinkley became, improbably enough, an advocate for women's rights. He was the only important broadcaster of his day to champion the American wife—she who "like the hart panteth for the running brook"—and talk about her sexual needs on the radio: "Don't get the impression that women are icebergs and are content with impotent husbands. I know of more families where the devil is to pay in fusses and temperamental sprees all due to the husband not being able to function properly. Many and many times, wives come to me and say, 'Doctor, my husband is no good.'"

Of course this was a way of hitting his target—men—from yet another angle; he knew that it was often someone with a rooting interest who got the patient on the train. Still, it bought him a lot of goodwill among the female population. Just like his promise that any woman who came to his clinic could "avail themselves to my years of study and practice and have their clitoris improved upon."

Businesswise it was all falling into place. He faced, however, one last threat.

Puritanism, famously defined by Mencken as "the haunting fear that someone, somewhere, may be happy," is as American as lighting out for the territory, and with the advent of radio the old war between the cowboys and the killjoys had broken out again. No sooner had Prohibition become the law of the land than broadcasting arrived, a miracle of fun and adventure that sent the puritans running right back to their storehouse of wet blankets. Along with the assigning of band waves came the U.S. government's quasilegal demand that all programming be high-minded and uplifting. As a result, orchestras played torpid "potted palm" music for hours on end. The infant NBC billed its first lineup of shows, with justice, as "the most pretentious broadcasting program ever presented." As for advertising, in 1924 more than 400 of the 526 radio stations then operating in America still accepted none. Radio czar Herbert Hoover, the secretary of commerce, declared it "inconceivable that we should allow so great a possibility for service to be drowned in advertiser chatter." Dr. Lee DeForest, whose invention of the three-element vacuum tube was a cornerstone of the infant technology, called the very thought of ads "a stench in the nostrils of the gods of the ionosphere." What commercials did go out over the air—for who could totally suppress them?—were expected to be short and sweet.

Dr. John Romulus Brinkley mooned the whole setup.

From the first he saw the future, and it was sales. A world-class huckster, he was also, according to one media historian, "the man who, perhaps, more than any other, foresaw the great potentialities of radio as an advertising medium." Quackery expert and Princeton University professor James Harvey Young agreed; to him, Brinkley was a morally repellent but shrewd individual who saw possibilities in radio advertising "to which most businessmen were blind."

This is not to say that corporate advertising was running in place. The new worship of science in the 1920s had touched many things (Nathan Leopold said he and Richard Loeb had killed Bobby Franks "in the interests of science"), and the ad business was no exception. A sea change had begun, a move away from "offering copy"—ads that presented the product factually, unadorned—to "selling copy," ads aimed at manufacturing desire in the undesiring breast. "Appeal to reason in your advertising," one up-to-date executive said, "and you appeal to about four percent of the human race."

It was a bit of a paradox, this new "science," based as it was on the circumvention of rational thought, but once stumbled upon it seemed blazingly obvious. Why had no one thought of it before? The answer was that somebody had: snake-oil salesmen. Targeting emotion was what medicine-show quacks and the big tonic manufacturers had been doing for decades. Now their huckstering, so shameless and so despised, had become the new template for corporate America.

The makers of Listerine were among the first to hit the pool.

Named for Sir Joseph Lister, the pioneer of antiseptic surgery, this hypermedicinal mixture had been genteelly promoted since the late nineteenth century chiefly to physicians as "the best antiseptic for both internal and external use," be it the treatment of venereal disease or "filling the cavity, during ovariotomy." But now Gerald Lambert, the son of the founder, saw a way to take his product from physicians' cabinets and drive it into America's cerebral cortex.

**You 5,000,000 women who want to get married:
How's Your Breath Today?**

Unleashed upon the country like a rat-borne plague, *halitosis* (a word derived from scary Latin) appeared overnight as the root cause of failed love affairs and smashed careers. Profits for Listerine's parent company jumped fortyfold. After that, affliction and marketing were America's hottest couple. In 1934 a publication called *Printer's Ink* totted up a list of physical ills created in whole or in part by advertising campaigns, including "acid indigestion, athlete's foot, body odor, calendar fear, coffee nerves, dry skin blight, folliculitis, intestinal fatigue, paralyzed pores, sandpaper bands, scalp crust, sneaker smell, and underarm offense."

Such was the new advertising of the 1920s: shameless hustling with a dusting of pseudoscience. Shameless, that is, in print ads. But American business failed for years to bring the same approach to the new world of radio. The fevered moralizing surrounding it was too daunting, the agility of thought demanded in boardrooms too great. One revolution at a time was enough.

While others shuffled forward then, Brinkley seized the day. He was the first to take product pitching out of the tents and town squares and put it on a national hookup. This would account for his fabulous success in the coming years: what he was selling *combined with* the hallucinatory force of his marketing. By 1924 an estimated 750 individuals and companies were promoting gland-rejuvenation treatments in the United States. But streaming out of Kansas on one of the strongest signals in the nation, Brinkley overpowered every competitor, promoting not just goat glands but the entire soup-to-nuts program of health-care offerings at the Brinkley Research Hospital.

"I want to digress now for a few minutes and carry you back to memory days. Those little memories that spring up along life's way like violets along a riverbank. In the heat of earthly struggles, as we are bewildered by vexing problems and saddened by testing trials, it is restful to fly to a nest of dreams made of tender vines and fragrant blooms plucked on a long journey down a trail of fond memories. . . ."

It wasn't all shoptalk. In interludes sometimes scripted, sometimes not, Doc Brinkley plucked the melic chords of yesteryear, and lulled by that trusted voice, his listeners, too, drifted and dreamed. "It is refreshing to wander back and sleep in the old cradle lighted by a flame in the chimney and rocked by the hand of an angel. . . ."

He poured so much syrup on the facts of his boyhood that some are now lost. But these in outline were his early years, these were the treasured hearts who reared him: his ex-Confederate, mountain doctor dad, who collapsed and died while making a house call; his mother ("the Bible was her library"), whose death scene pushed Little Nell out of bed; his sainted Aunt Sally . . .

Then, with a benediction for his listeners, he yielded the microphone. Even the doctor couldn't talk for fifteen and a half hours a day, and besides, no one comes to a medicine show just for the tonic. To keep folks tuned in he featured a grab bag of entertainment, including live military bands, French lessons, astrologers, gospel quartets, the Tell-Me-a-Story Lady, and Hawaiian songs of farewell. Country music, too: within a year of its radio debut, a performance by Fiddlin' John Carson over WSB in Atlanta, Brinkley was paying top dollar to recruit champion fiddle player Uncle Bob Larkin and other stars, and launching discoveries of his own like Roy Faulkner, aka the Lonesome Cowboy. A short man with a tall pompadour and easy grin, Faulkner sang the old songs in a sunny voice like Gene Autry's and became Brinkley's most famous house musician. He and the rest of the KFKB troupe—Zapata's Novelty Troubadours, Albert Fenoglio and his accordion, the Harmony Boys, et al.—performed in a studio furnished like a large late-Victorian parlor, and listeners had an open invitation to drop by and share the good times. "You could go in there and sit in that studio and watch some of the best entertainment in the world," recalled goat-gland daddy Stittsworth who, like other farmers, also came to depend on the station's grain and livestock reports.

Not only did Brinkley speak to the common people but he also spoke for them, and he established KFKB as the trumpet of small-town pride. Thanks to battery-powered receivers, he could reach into the most isolated homes. In the dead of night, when everyone else had left the studio, he consoled the desolate as they lay awake.

"I have here a letter from a farmer, a tiller of the soil who has given himself without stint, with his simple generosity that the great cities may live . . ."

When his transmitter burned down, he built a better one.

On Sundays he gave sermons lifted from other people.

19

Overseas, the price of chimpanzees was up 600 percent. That is, if you could find one at all: there was growing fear that they might be wiped out by a mad confluence of hunters, clothing designers (who craved the fur), and gland enthusiasts. Dr. Maurice Lebon, "noted French savant," declared that unless steps were taken at once, this incomparable rejuvenation technique might become tragically moot.

To prevent this catastrophe, Serge Voronoff himself contributed one hundred thousand francs to the Pasteur Institute's emergency monkey farm in French West Africa. He also founded his own chimp-breeding center on the Italian Riviera, set on a hillside beneath his baronial chateau. Standing at the window with a glass of vodka (source of the Voronoff family fortune), he could enjoy the sunset music of primates rising from the woods below. Some said success had gone to his head, but if so, had he not earned it? In October 1922 he had been booed off the stage while attempting to address the French Academy of Medicine in Paris. Now he was writing the *rejuvenation* entry for the Encyclopedia Britannica. Oohed and aahed over everywhere he went, he and his young American wife roved across Europe from spa to casino to grand hotel, fixtures of the international set, from which he increasingly drew his clientele. With charitable exceptions, his minimum fee was five thousand dollars. Before implanting them he wrapped the monkey glands in silk.

Challenges still confronted him, one of the greatest being the level of liveliness in the average chimpanzee. "It is not possible to get the ape onto the table while conscious," Voronoff wrote, "as even the gentlest subjects fight desperately [any] attempt to tie their limbs. They are extremely suspicious and, in order to anesthetize them, it is necessary to resort to strategy." By this he meant a double-chambered cage he designed himself, rather like the air-lock system found in submarines. An ordinary wire pen opened onto a short hallway that led to the solid-walled "Anesthetizing Box." But time was of the essence. Once gassed, the animal had to be gotten "out of the cage and onto the operating table . . . before he is sufficiently recovered to get his teeth into the hands of those who control him."

Along with his chimp-to-man practice, Voronoff also began transplanting (à la Mrs. Stittsworth) monkey ovaries into women. This led to a one-off in the reverse direction: implanting a woman's ovary in a chimpanzee. The monkey, named Nora, was then inseminated with human sperm. (The only thing that produced was a novel, Félicien Champsaur's *Nora, la guenon devenue femme—Nora, the Monkey Turned Woman*—which recounted the adventures of the demidemoiselle in the Folies Bergère.) Voronoff ventured, too, into the horse-racing world. In December 1923, his attempts to rejuvenate an ancient former champion named Ayala with an equine-gland transplant failed when the horse died thrashing under the anesthetic. Soon after, though, he tried another, reportedly with better results: "The horse is in very good condition and within several weeks will be put into training for racing." Along the way *Scientific American* praised his progress, and testimonials appeared in the press. Arthur Evelyn Liardet, an elderly client from England, invited reporters to squeeze his rejuvenated bicep. "Voronoff told me," he said, "that when I again felt myself growing old he would repeat the operation, and that he could perform it in all three times. That ought to take me to the age of 150."

If Voronoff had his Liardet, the rivalrous Dr. Steinach could point to his own happy Brit. A London businessman named Alfred Wilson underwent the Austrian's protovasectomy and was so delighted with the results—he felt twenty years younger, he said—that he booked the Royal Albert Hall to lecture on his transformation. On the day before he was scheduled to speak Wilson experienced chest pains. These were laughingly attributed to his new habit of pounding himself on the chest like Tarzan, till he went into full cardiac arrest and died.

There was no room for truth, however, now that fantasy had booked the hotel. Steinach and his "vasoligation" breakthrough were the toast of Vienna. Compared with Voronoff's, his claims were slightly less sensational. "We cannot . . . perform the comic opera bouffe of transmuting an old hag into a giddy young damsel . . . ," he warned. "But, under certain conditions, we can stretch the span of . . . usefulness, and enable the patient to recapture the raptures, if not the giddiness, of youth." Senility, he flatly declared, was "reversible."

Sigmund Freud was "Steinached" in November 1923. Fighting oral cancer, the sixty-seven-year-old Freud hoped the operation would at least keep it at bay and restore his zest for life. Whether he felt any benefit from the procedure was disputed ever after. Decades later Dr. Harry Benjamin, a sometime colleague of Steinach's, claimed that Freud told him personally he was "very satisfied with the result. His general health and vitality had improved and he also thought that the malignant growth of his jaw had been favorably influenced. 'Don't talk about it as long as I am alive,' he said to me on parting." Others, however, said the great man thought it was worthless.

Either way Freud stayed silent, but a book called *Black Oxen* by Gertrude Atherton made Steinach a star in America. The nation's most popular novel of 1923, outselling even Anita Loos's *Gentlemen Prefer Blondes,* Atherton's tale turned on Steinach's real-life rejuvenation treatment for women. In the novel young Mary Ogden leaves the United States for Austria. Decades later the mysterious and equally young Madame Zattiany, visiting from Europe, knocks New York society off its pins by revealing that she is, yes, Mary Ogden rejuvenated— thanks to Dr. Steinach, who has dosed her ovaries with radiation. When a journalist named Clavering falls in love with her, he finds himself lost in a forest of metaphysics:

> It might be the greatest discovery of all time, but . . . it would be hard on the merely young. The mutual hatreds of capital and labor would sink into insignificance before the antagonism between authentic youth and age inverted. . . . The threat of overpopulation—for man's architectonic powers were restored if not woman's; to say nothing of his prolonged sojourn—would at last rouse the law-makers to the imperious necessity of eugenics, birth control, sterilization of the unfit, and the expulsion of undesirable races.

Here the author, Miss Atherton (who had herself undergone eight sessions of ovary radiation), nicely put her finger on some of the stupendous problems the specter of mass rejuvenation raised, and which many found sincerely frightening. Eugenics, the notion of improving animals and plants through particularized breeding techniques, was already a hot branch of science found in many textbooks, including the one used by John Scopes to teach evolution. Eugenics societies sponsored popular "Beautiful Baby" and "Fitter Family" contests at county fairs. That was its happy face. But its proponents were also the driving force behind legislation like Virginia's racial purity law (mocked by Morris Fishbein in an article for Mencken), and the prospect of introducing glands into the mix had the totalitarians on full alert. Who should be allowed to rejuvenate themselves? Not the retarded certainly, or the insane or criminals or anyone else with "bad heredity"—or, come to think of it, most "normal" people either, since according to the Eugenics Society only 4 percent of America's children were "high-grade person[s] who will have the ability to do creative work and be fit for leadership." The price of perfection was eternal vigilance, or the world would fill up with idiots and Dorian Grays.

Business likewise was scrambling to prepare for that hallelujah morning that mass rejuvenation might produce. Insurance companies especially were all at sea, since it threatened to make nonsense of their actuarial tables. In 1923 author and gland enthusiast George F. Corners reported on a meeting of New York City underwriters where the potential effects of gland science on "life insurance, disability clauses, etc., was discussed with much animation. Provisions for old age, pensions, etc., will be subjected to substantial modifications," though what those modifications might be none could yet say. While they agonized, a European insurance firm took the leap, refusing to pay an old-age pension to a retired businessman who had undergone a monkey-gland transplant, on the grounds that he was no longer old. "We have learned that last fall you underwent an operation according to the method of Dr. Voronoff," the letter stated, "and, consequently, it follows that you are younger today than you were when you signed the contract with us. In view of this fundamental change we find ourselves obliged to cancel the contract with you." The policyholder sued.

For many months Dr. Max Thorek had been toiling on the rooftop with his menagerie. But somehow despite the thrilling results others reported, every one of his own gland experiments had ended in failure.

One Sunday morning several of his chimps escaped, reassembling for reasons unknown at the nearby Church of Our Lady of the Lake. Thorek rushed to the scene. "[U]ntil the Scopes trial came along the following year," he later wrote, "it was the most dramatic collision of monkeys and the Christian faith Americans had ever seen—at least Father Denison and his slack-jawed congregation, who were left queasily wondering forever after: Why?

"I have far too much respect for all religions to be so sacrilegious as to place on record the actions of those monkeys. It suffices to say that a Rabelais or a Voltaire or a Swift would have leaped upon that incident, and added another chapter to the classics of satire. As far as I was concerned, it was the end."

20

In the summer of 1925, H. L. Mencken went south to Dayton, Tennessee, to cover the Scopes trial, that epic clash between Darwinians and Christian fundamentalists. A local schoolteacher, John Scopes, was charged with teaching the theory of evolution to children, and he stood now like another Galileo in the dock. Clarence Darrow, the famed defense attorney, had come from Chicago to represent him; the old-time religionists were championed by three-time presidential candidate William Jennings Bryan. To Mencken the prosecution was a thrilling display of ignorance on parade, and the town itself a wilderness of monkeys.

Together with Fishbein, Mencken had recently produced a major exposé on faith healers, and between court sessions he mailed his collaborator this flyer from the scene:

COMING! COMING!

To

DAYTON TENNESSEE

During the Trial of the Infidel Scopes

ELMER CHUBB, L.L.D., D.D.

FUNDAMENTALIST AND MIRACLE WORKER

MIRACLES PERFORMED ON THE PUBLIC SQUARE!

Dr. Chubb will allow himself to be bitten by any poisonous snake, scorpion, gila monster, or other reptile. He will also drink any poison brought to him.

In demonstration of the words of our Lord and Saviour
Jesus Christ, as found in the 16th Chapter of the
Gospel of St. Mark:

"And these signs shall follow them that believe: in my
name shall they cast out devils, they shall speak with
new tongues; they shall take up serpents, and if they
drink any deadly thing it shall in no wise hurt them;
they shall lay hands on the sick and
they shall recover."

Public demonstration of healing, casting out
devils, and prophesying, Dr. Chubb will also
preach in Aramaic, Hebrew, Greek, Latin, Coptic,
Egyptian, and in the lost tongues of the Etruscans
and the Hittites.

TESTIMONIALS; All favorable but one:
With my own eyes I saw Dr. Chubb swallow
cyanide of potassium.
—WILLIAM JENNINGS BRYAN,
Christian Statesman

Dr. Chubb simply believes the word of God,
and his power follows.
—REV. J. FRANK NORRIS.

I was possessed of devils, and Dr. Chubb cast them
out of me. Glory to God.
—MAGDALENA RAYBACK
RFD 3, Duncan Grove, Mich.

When under the spell of divine inspiration Dr. Chubb
speaks Coptic as fluently as if it were his mother tongue.
As to Etruscan I cannot say.

—PROF. ADDISON BLAKESLEY, Professor of ancient
languages at Valparaiso University, Ind.

Chubb is a fake. I can mix a cyanide cocktail that will make
him turn up his toes in thirty seconds.
—H. L. MENCKEN

SPECIAL NOTICE:
Dr. Chubb has never pretended that he had power to **RAISE
THE DEAD.** The Bible shows that only the Saviour and the
Twelve Apostles had that power.

*Free will offering, dedicated to the enforcement of the anti-
evolution law.*

It was a joke. Mencken and Edgar Lee Masters (of Schlogl's and
Spoon River Anthology fame) had composed it together. Then
Mencken hired a boy to pass out a thousand copies around town and
waited to see what would happen. What happened was nothing. The
town was already crawling with the real thing.

As for Fishbein, he had just moved to Blackstone Avenue, along
with his wife, Anna, and their three children, into a house principally
designed by Frank Lloyd Wright: an elegant eight rooms, every window a different shape, some with a view of Lake Michigan. While the
Medical Mussolini, Medical Midas, and Drugstore Dumas (his enemies never tired of euphony) thrived on war in his professional life,
he insisted on domestic tranquillity—which is not to say he relaxed.
Fishbein flung himself into fatherhood as he did everything else,
teaching his daughter Marjorie to shoot craps in the backseat of his
chauffeured Cadillac, and carting her off at her request to a performance by Gypsy Rose Lee. "We saw Jack Dempsey box," his other
daughter, Barbara, recalled. "We also ran with Daddy every time we
heard a fire engine."

The big new house went along with a big promotion: Fishbein

had been appointed editor in chief of *JAMA*, the job for which he had long been groomed. He started off with two full-time secretaries, then hired a third, and quickly solidified his image as all-knowing, all-seeing demiurge of the AMA—or as a tour guide accidentally called it, "the American Fishbein Association." Churning out books and articles at the rate of fifteen thousand words a week, he turned *JAMA* from a minor trade organ into a potent social-policy voice, traveled incessantly (a reporter claimed that Fishbein "flies so much he sometimes finds himself reaching for a seat belt when he sits in an ordinary chair"), and delivered 130 speeches a year. Inspirational orator or indefatigable gasbag? Reasonable minds might differ, but as spokesman for a hundred thousand doctors with a united opinion on nothing, most counted him a success, less as a politician than as a force of nature.

Everywhere he scorned claims of a fountain of youth, whether homegrown or European. "There is no such thing as artificial rejuvenation as advertised by Brinkley and other such quacks," he said. ". . . [I]t is the acme of foolishness for old men to spend their money . . . trying to defeat nature." As for the "Steinachian miracle," he pointed out that vasectomies had been performed before the Austrian ever appeared on the scene, and "in not one of the hundreds of cases of cutting the ducts reported previous to the time of Steinach did any of the meticulous surgeons . . . mention any restoration of youthful vigor." Though most scientists and editors still treated the topic with at least cautious respect, Fishbein refused to publish articles in *JAMA* supporting it.

He still found time to moonlight for Mencken. Unfortunately, the collaboration required that Fishbein make the occasional pilgrimage to Baltimore, which always seemed to land him in dens of iniquity.

Mencken liked to call alcohol "the father and mother of joy," and Prohibition had set him to bootlegging on an almost Caponean scale. First he had sold his car to stock up on "the best wines and liquors I could find," stashing them in a basement vault with a skull and crossbones on the door and a sign threatening intruders with chlorine gas. He also conducted experiments in homebrew involving automobile gloves and "fearful explosions." As a drinker Fishbein wasn't nearly in the same class, but whenever he came to town Mencken carted him off to clubs. "The scene of the little German band will always be vivid in my memory," Fishbein wrote to him in January 1925. "On Sunday, I found purple specks under my eye, and in the afternoon the blood spots began to appear on the cornea." Graciously he added, "I am quite sure this was not due to the baccardi." After his next visit, however, he informed Mencken he had "returned to Chicago spotted like a leopard. It is alleged that it was caused by the fluids imbibed at the Italian's place in Baltimore." For a time he avoided the city.

Were they friends? Yes, but how close that friendship was may lie in the eye of the beholder. Mencken had the more complicated heart. Any statement about his attitude toward Jews is contradicted by the evidence, but his view of Fishbein is at least partly contained in this diary entry, written when they had known each other more than twenty years: "[T]here is a shrewd Jew in him at bottom, and I am inclined to believe that his services to American medicine have been extremely valuable."

21

The summer of the Scopes trial, Dr. and Mrs. Brinkley traveled to Italy. After sampling the pleasures of Milan they made a short trip south to the ancient university town of Pavia, where the roster of graduates included Christopher Columbus.

Keen on shoring up his credentials after the diploma-mill crisis, Brinkley had come to Europe in search of honorary degrees. Dublin rebuffed him, London and Glasgow, too. But in the charming backwater of Pavia, officials knew less about him. His owlish veneer, his adroit flattery, his offer of an endowment—all impressed the unworldly elders of the university's medical school. And then he fed them: consommé frappé à l'Impératrice, vol au vent à la Toulousaine, flan de légumes à la Financière, glace à la Napolitaine, along with bottles of Bardolino, Barolo, and Piper Heidsieck champagne. . . . The doctor even hired an orchestra to accompany the banquet with mellow offerings by Mendelssohn, Puccini, and Irving Berlin. He got his degree.

All the while he had been following the news from the States, and one story in particular fired his imagination. On his return home, he took the lessons of the Scopes trial and wove them into a new business plan.

Christianity was back in the headlines anyway. America's bestselling nonfiction book of 1925 and 1926 was Bruce Barton's *The Man Nobody Knows: A Discovery of Jesus.* Its premise—which would no doubt be just as commercial today—was that Christ was the world's first great business executive because "he took twelve men from the bottom ranks and forged them into an organization that conquered the world." Along with being a champion service provider, Jesus was also "the greatest advertiser" of his era. "Take any one of the parables, no matter which—you will find that it exemplifies all the principles on which advertising text books are written. . . . First of all they are marvelously condensed, as all good advertising must be. . . . Sincerity glistened like sunshine through every sentence [Christ] uttered. . . . Finally he knew the necessity of repetition and practiced it."

For some time Brinkley had been noticing the resemblance between himself and the Son of God. (His review of Barton's book: "That seems to be my life all over.") But the Scopes trial affected him, publicly at least, like a bracing full-body baptism. That fall on the radio he spread the word and shared the rapture more freely than ever before. His self-reinvention flowered forth in this exquisite puff piece in the *New York Evening Journal:*

Preaches Fundamentalism—Practices Goat Gland Science
How a Famous Surgeon Combines Old-Time Religion
and Newfangled Operations on a Strange
Medico-Gospel Farm

"Meet the most unusual scientist-fundamentalist in the whole world, Dr. John R. Brinkley of Milford, Kansas."

A précis of his heroic career followed, from his "daring experiments" as an "AEF veterinary surgeon" during the Great War up through his honorary degree in Pavia—just the third time in history, the doctor revealed, that the university had granted such an honor, the previous recipients being Napoleon and Michelangelo.

"Back in the States," the article continued:

Brinkley found a storm brewing in his home state, Tennessee [*sic*]. The great Scopes trial was in process of incubation. The returning scientist, himself a Tennessean [*sic*], saw and sympathized with the mountaineers' efforts to keep their beloved religion untouched by scientific fingers. Perhaps some hidden mental echo of his boyhood in that region [*sic*] awoke within him the latest sparks of devotional fervor. Perhaps the white-hot oratory of the late William Jennings Bryan struck a response in his heart.

Whatever the cause, Brinkley opened his hands to fundamentalism. He converted his spacious grounds at Milford into a glorified camp-meeting ground. . . . Thus soul-saving and bodily repairing went hand in hand under the keen eye of one of the best scientists and firmest 'believers' on the globe.

Minnie is quoted describing their new outdoor theater where "moral and religious pictures are shown to remind [people] of the Greatest Man ever known."

There were many photographs.

**PREACHES GOSPEL Dr. Charles Draper,
Pastor of the Brinkley Institute,
Who Doesn't Believe in Scientific
Evolution**

**SUNDAY SCHOOL CHILDREN on the
Playground at Milford, Kansas, Where
Rigid Fundamentalism Is Taught, Despite
the Adjacency of Dr. Brinkley's Gland
Hospital Activities**

**BRINKLEY HOLDS BILLY, First
'Goat-Gland Baby'**

How young Charles Darwin Mellinger, the town's second "goat-gland baby," fared under the new regime is unrecorded. But as a result of this master class in propaganda, Brinkley's mail jumped to three thousand letters a day.

Andy Whitebeck of Council Bluffs, Iowa, was among the many

thousands of KFKB listeners whose hearts were stirred by the doctor's high endeavor. Whitebeck had longed for one of Brinkley's four-phase compound gland operations, but he and his wife were barely scraping by. The only thing they owned of any value was their house. Now, as if answering a call to prayer, they mortgaged their home, and Whitebeck made the trip to Brinkley's clinic.

There he met another patient, farmer Joseph Fritz from Nebraska. "Andy told me all about it," Fritz remembered years later.

He said he and his wife talked it over and agreed that Brinkley was such a good Christian man, he preached such lovely sermons over the radio every Sunday, when he found out how poor Andy was and how he could raise only $550 by mortgaging his home, he'd surely operate on Andy for that, and maybe, like the Good Samaritan in the Bible, he'd do it for nothing, and say to Andy, "Go on home and give the money back to your wife and lift the mortgage on your little home and God bless you both."

But Brinkley was not that kind of a Christian. When Andy got there with only $550 Brinkley wouldn't touch him. He'd have to raise $750 or go home without an operation.

I never felt so sorry for anyone in all my life as I did for Andy as he stood there, weeping like a child. He wanted that operation so bad so he could go back home and to his old job.

Then Minnie Brinkley (who liked to describe her role at the clinic as "counseling, collecting and good will") stepped in. "[She] told him he'd just have to raise the other $200, and they worked on his fears, made him think the goat glands were the only things that could save him and make him young and strong again, and Andy didn't know where to turn for the money. With tears in his eyes he begged Brinkley to take his note for $200 and he'd pay it, little by little, out of his wages as he earned them." Brinkley refused. Finally, said Fritz, "Mrs. Brinkley wrote to the firm Andy worked for, and she got a written agreement from it that it would send so much of Andy's wages to her each week till the two hundred dollars was paid, and then [they] operated on him, and sent him back to his mortgaged home and his wages also mortgaged for months."

The operation was useless, Fritz added. Whitebeck wrote and told him he was "much worse than he was before Brinkley worked on him. . . . Brinkley merely operated on his pocketbook." As for Fritz, he felt lucky to get out alive.

Unfortunately the better the publicity machine, the more likely it is to reach the wrong people.

When Dr. Max Thorek, Brinkley's former teacher and longtime foe, read about the Pavia degree, he indignantly cabled the university to protest. Then Fishbein got into the act, and the two pelted the Italian government and the school with choice facts about their honoree. It worked: the degree was personally revoked by Benito Mussolini.

Brinkley claimed the diploma for the rest of his life.

22

Walking back toward the sanitarium after visiting Sandburg again, Eugene Debs collapsed on the sidewalk. Within the hour Morris Fishbein's telephone rang. He was astonished to learn that Debs, whom he had not seen in more than four years, had left word that if his life was ever in danger, Fishbein was the doctor he wanted.

Since he wasn't a practicing physician, he brought two other doctors with him to Debs's bedside. But the great socialist was past saving. "Mr. Debs . . . was clearly the victim of malnutrition," Fishbein later wrote. The subject "lay in bed barely breathing. . . . Confronted with this situation, the healers of the naturopathic sanatorium had attempted to [apply] diathermy or electrical heat. Perhaps because of the unconsciousness of the patient, he had suffered burns which were visible on the skin at the points of application of the electrodes." When these failed, attendants injected cactus dissolved in water—"an old eclectic remedy"—and then digitalis, too little and then too much. Within hours Debs was dead.

That night in October 1926 left Fishbein seething. The year before he had produced a book, *Medical Follies*, which itemized a slew of frauds, fads, and delusions. Now he wrote another, *New Medical Follies* (1927), a fresh catalogue of quackeries which, said the *New York Times*, he "variously impales, flays, or neatly spits and roasts in the fires of his indignation." Among them were food faddists and weight-reduction extremists like Lindlahr, who he believed had killed Debs.

There was a chapter on rejuvenation, too. Voronoff and Steinach's work was again dissected and trampled on, although Fishbein presented the men themselves as more benighted than venal. Dr. Brinkley, whom Fishbein had always viewed as a lower form of life, was not mentioned—not until a few months later, in January 1928, when the editor first took public aim at "the Burbank of Humanity" in a broadside devoted exclusively to him.

Unambiguously entitled "John R. Brinkley—Quack, The Commercial Possibilities of Goat-Gland Grafting," the *JAMA* article detailed the ins and outs of the goat racket, and it broke news as well. Fishbein used the resources of his "fun department," the AMA's Bureau of Investigation, to unearth the story of Brinkley's early days as an electromedic jailbird and lay it before the public for the first time.

Or at least a sliver of the public. As an Illinois doctor wrote Fishbein when the article appeared: "The trouble is that we [M.D.s] who already know, read it, and the poor devils who should be warned, do not subscribe to the *JAMA*." Well aware of the problem, Fishbein took the rare step of reprinting his exposé as a pamphlet and distributing it by the thousands. But even then he was shouting into the wind. The kind of mass outrage he could have mustered in a later era was a Sisyphean task in the 1920s, when "the media" had yet to be invented and even the big cities were still small towns. Scalawags benefited hugely from this parochialism. In Massachusetts, a self-styled forensics authority named A. J. Hamilton, caught red-handed trying to switch gun barrels during the trial of Sacco and Vanzetti, had a thriving career for years afterward as an expert witness in other states. As for Brinkley, he had the massive advantage of his radio station. To legions of listeners like Alexander Ekblon, he *was* the media.

Ekblon's wife, Rose, was dying of colon cancer. Military surgeons at Fort Riley, where he worked as a coal shoveler, told him her case was hopeless. "But I loved my wife very much," he said later. "I would have given my own life to save her if I could, and . . . a man in my place, about to see the wife he loves drift out on the tide, will grasp at any straw." In his anguish he turned to Brinkley, who told him there was still a chance. Ekblon "scraped around and borrowed" the money for an operation, Brinkley performed it, and Rose Ekblon died the next day. The Milford Messiah demanded and collected his $350 fee.

Meanwhile goat-gland patients kept streaming into his medical casino. Nine days after surgery, housepainter John Homback was taken ill in the St. Louis train station on his way home to New Jersey. Doctors at the Missouri Baptist Hospital discovered he was in the primary stages of lockjaw. Despite the gangrenous incisions on his scrotum, Homback insisted through clenched teeth that Brinkley had done "wonderful" work, while a Dr. Mayes flooded Homback with antitetanus serum, both subcutaneous and intravenous. "The patient seemed to respond to the treatment," Mayes wrote. "His spasms had been greatly relieved and his jaws were not locked, as he showed me how he could open his mouth as soon as he heard my voice. About three hours later the patient took a severe convulsion and died." His stricken son, Carl Homback, railed at Brinkley's butchery: "I hope somebody strings him up." But the law still couldn't touch him.

Instead he grew and prospered. In 1928 Brinkley had his next eureka moment, an inspiration that would earn him millions. What was this great insight? His purported discovery of "a relationship of cause and effect between the [goat] gland operation and the reduction in the size of the prostate."

In other words, here was a way to use the same operation to appeal to a vast new clientele. Or—another thought—what if he also offered to shrink the prostate without surgery? Just how he would accomplish this feat remained unclear, at least in his mailings; all his customers had to know was that the prostate didn't have to be removed nearly as often as the "Amateur Meatcutters Association" (his sarcastic name for the AMA) claimed it did. This breakthrough, it went without saying, was "a crowning achievement . . . a service to humanity that will live for centuries to come."

Every innovator knows that zone where the ideas come in bunches. Soon he would have a third. And that scheme, wholly different from the rest, was destined to become the most popular and profitable of his career. It was aimed, ironically enough, at women.

23

Ten cents straight will be charged for all obituary notices to all business men who do not advertise while living. Delinquent subscribers will be charged fifteen cents per line for an obituary notice. Advertisers and cash subscribers will receive as good a send-off as we are capable of writing, without any charge whatsoever. Better send in your subscription, as the hog cholera is abroad in the land.

— ALTOONA (KANSAS) TRIBUNE, JANUARY 1928

On warm-weather weekends holidaymakers descended on the grounds of the Brinkley Research Hospital, spreading picnic lunches on the grass, playing tag, and feeding the famous goats. Roy Faulkner, the Lonesome Cowboy, squeezed through crowds so thick "there wasn't room to walk" as he moved about playing his guitar. Folks were tickled to death to see him in the flesh, and their other radio favorites, too.

Of course the face most eagerly sought was Dr. Brinkley's. Along with their panfried chicken and rhubarb pie, some of these day-trippers brought ailments, some severe, some—well, you couldn't always tell. A fever, a scratch, sometimes the littlest thing could turn around and kill you, so there were always some panicky people in the crowd. Plus the chronic cases hobbling around or laid out half-paralyzed as if they'd just staggered into Lourdes. Whenever Brinkley did make an appearance, he could hardly take a step without somebody grabbing his coat.

No doctor would have enjoyed that, of course, but Brinkley liked it less than most because he hated giving free advice. Still, he was caught between a rock and a hard place. He couldn't very well hide out when five hundred people came to call. On the other hand, all the whining and pleading was driving him crazy.

Then, as if from the head of Zeus, sprang the great idea. He called it *Medical Question Box*.

It worked like this. Listeners were invited to write to him describing a medical problem, their own or that of someone they knew. Brinkley would read some of the letters, diagnose each case, and suggest treatment—all on the radio. Launched in early 1928, *Medical Question Box* was a sensation. Each day *MQB* secretary Ruth Athey and eight assistants swam through the mail, almost all of it from women—women anxious over their own health, their husbands', their children's, their neighbors'—and plucked from this sea of suffering about seventy-five letters to pass along to the boss. The rest were thrown away. Brinkley glanced through the finalists and used what he liked.

Diagnosing the invisible, drugging the unseen: taking on the complex role of conservative fundamentalist visionary, Brinkley opened new vistas in healing which, he predicted, would one day make trips to the doctor obsolete. Eventually thousands of physicians would follow his lead, operating not with an old-fashioned scalpel but with a "radio knife," one which "does not burn or cut." On he went, offering counsel and comfort freely—but anyone who thought it was free wasn't paying attention.

A woman writes to Brinkley about her six-year-old daughter who is complaining of cramps. After reading the letter on air, Brinkley tells the mother and the rest of the audience, "I think she is wormy. Ask for Prescription 94 for worms. In regard to yourself, you had your appendix taken out. You are going to get into a little trouble later on. My advice is number 61 and stay on it for about ten years."

To a query from Dresden, Kansas: "Probably he has gallstones. No, I don't mean that, I mean kidney stones. My advice to you is to put him on Prescription No. 80 and 50 for men, also 64. I think that he will be a whole lot better. Also drink a lot of water."

The money was in the drugs. In a burst of enterprise he roped together about five hundred midwestern drugstores into the Brinkley Pharmaceutical Association, shrewdly installing as president a Topeka druggist who was brother-in-law to the state attorney general. The doctor then supplied them all with a line of stratospherically overpriced medications, some off the shelf, some of his own devising, all smartly repackaged with numbers instead of names to enhance their mystique and conceal their ingredients. With rare exceptions he prescribed nothing else on *Medical Question Box*. And here was the beauty part: every diagnosis he made reached not just the letter writer but hundreds, thousands of other listeners who, while they drank in details of the case on the radio, often realized they were crawling with the same symptoms. The pharmacists kicked back one dollar to Brinkley on each jar sold (at about six times normal retail) and kept the rest.

From pinworms to lumbago, from heart disease to clammy hands, no disease was too large or too small for *Medical Question Box*. With those treatments that required preparation—the ones that weren't pills from Parke-Davis with the labels switched—Brinkley often took great pains with quality control. Some of the down-home stuff he apparently believed in. "Prescription No. 7," he advised his pharmacists, "is an old time-honored itch medicine. Equal parts of black gunpowder, sulphur and hog lard, or any Vaseline or greasy base. The secret of its results is in its application. Instruct the patient to go home, take a hot bath and dry thoroughly, grease themselves from head to foot with this: put on a union-suit, stockings, and soft cloth gloves and go to bed. Grease for the second and third nights without bathing, wearing the same underclothing and sleeping in the same bed. On the 4th day take a good hot bath, boil the bedding and clothing worn; and if you have been careful the itch is gone." Remarkably enough, all sales were *not* final. "Always make a refund on any prescription where the patient is not 100% pleased, and charge me up with the refund," he wrote. "I want 100% satisfaction." Where lesser charlatans would have gone for the quick buck, Brinkley always saw the big picture. For every complainer there would be five new customers coming through the door because he was so honest.

24

On the afternoon of November 2, 1929, Happy Harry pulled up in front of the clinic with another raddled busload of new recruits. Among them was John Zahner, a sixty-five-year-old fruit grower from Lenexa, Kansas. A cadaverous 6'2", with hair like a hedge, Zahner was a longtime listener to KFKB. Like most farmers he was not an impulsive man, but after two years that unwearying hypnotist's voice had eaten away his resistance. His wife, too, had been pestering him to get goat glands. So here he was at last, embarked on what he regarded as "this great and confusing adventure."

As usual Minnie was there to welcome the new arrivals, her smile sunnier than ever. After more than ten years of trying, the Brinkleys finally had a child of their own; Johnny Boy, age two, stood beside her now clutching her dress. The doctor had been at pains to tell the press that goat glands were not involved.

Along a plush strip of Oriental carpet the men trooped down the hall to the herd room, where each was issued a bathrobe, nightgown, and slippers—except that Zahner got no slippers because there weren't any big enough. A doctor pointed at his feet and laughed. From somewhere in the building came the sound of a man's voice, loud and peeved. Apparently one of last week's patients hadn't been cleared out yet, and someone wasn't happy about it.

Staff doctors now took the men off for individual exams. Zahner drew Brinkley's one-eared chief assistant, H. D. Osborn, who took him into a small room and checked him over for about twenty minutes.

Osborn wasn't the reassuring sort. Above his dark little mustache were the eyes of a very patient lizard. Producing a sharp instrument, he made a gash on Zahner's forearm. Then, musing over the wound, Osborn told him that such rapid blood loss was proof of a serious condition. It signaled that Zahner's prostate was so swollen it was now (in Osborn's words) "as big as my fist," and that the full four-phase compound goat-gland operation was imperative.

Zahner balked. He had promised his wife he would have this done, or something like it, but he was confused now and scared. It was all happening too fast. Perhaps he could start with one of those cheaper nonsurgical prostate reductions Dr. Brinkley had mentioned on the radio.

No, no, no, Osborn said, bandaging the arm. He needed "the works."

But first he should rest. An aide took Zahner away to his room, all goose down and chintz, with Brinkley's soft drone coming from the radio. Soon Minnie tapped at the door. His operation had been scheduled for the morning, she said. It was for the good of himself and his family. The farmer said he was thinking it over.

For the next couple of hours he lay in a brown study. He didn't like the feel of the place at all—but what if these people were right? And his wife was counting on him to go through with it.

Counting on him, in fact, more than he ever dreamed. Back home in Lenexa, the former Minerva Kleer, thirty-seven, couldn't wait for her husband to have the operation because she couldn't wait for him to be dead.

It's unclear whether Mrs. Zahner had looked into Brinkley's track record herself and come away optimistic. But sometime before her husband left for Milford she consulted a Kansas City fortune-teller, who told her that he wouldn't live out the year. Rather, he would return home after his goat-gland operation and drop dead in a lumberyard, leaving her a rich widow. Now, with her husband off at Brinkley's, she was already having the house redecorated.

Zahner fell asleep, missed dinner, and woke up late in the evening. From down the hall he could hear the low voices and hushed laughter of the night staff. His eyes rested on a picture on the opposite wall, a painting of a shepherdess with her bonnet and crook. At this hour, in these shadows, she bore an unhappy resemblance to the Grim Reaper.

He fell asleep again.

At two in the morning he came awake. A figure stood at his bedside. He flailed up onto his elbows.

I have news, the specter said.

He peered: Minnie Brinkley again. She was holding a clipboard with his still-unsigned authorization. Minnie told him that further tests on his blood had shown he was a "borderline case," and she left no doubt what borderline she was talking about. Uremic poisoning had already set in, and if he didn't have the four-phase compound operation immediately, he would not live out the month. If he did, he would be cured in three days. "She scared me," he said later. "I believe I never would have signed it if she had come to me in daylight, but at that uncanny hour of night, with the sick men all limping up and down the halls, light flickering, examinations going on . . . I signed."

25

With members of the Brinkley Pharmaceutical Association reporting sales jumps as high as seventy-five dollars a day, the trade magazine *Midwestern Druggist* swooned: "The results that [Brinkley] has been able to produce . . . have been phenomenal . . . more like a fairy tale than real happenings in a modern business." Even ethically minded pharmacists found the money hard to resist. At least until the reports of trouble started coming in.

Dr. H. W. Gilley of Ottawa, Kansas, was brought to the bedside of a mailman on the edge of death. "I found the patient profoundly collapsed," Gilley reported, "his countenance ghastly, icy cold, pulse-less, and apparently dying from some great shock. Upon my question as to what had happened he whispered: 'I took some of Brinkley's medicine.'"

The doctor examined the bottle: Brinkley's No. 50, liver medicine, price $3.50. Aside from being worth about seventy-five cents, as later tests proved, Gilley found the effect of this No. 50 to have been "so drastic upon the patient as to produce enormous cholera-like gripings and actions and vomiting, causing a tearing open of [an] old ulcer and violent hemorrhage. . . . [T]he vomiting and intense pain continuing, X-ray pictures were taken, showing the pyloric orifice about one and a half inches to be nearly closed, and it will soon be imperative to make a new opening by attaching the bowel to the lower margin of the stomach."

As other patients suffered similar disasters, a surgeon named

Dawson spoke for thousands of physicians in this letter to a Kansas newspaper:

> It is not in the hope of increasing our business or of putting down a competitor that we are trying to strangle Brinkley. But it is because Brinkley is an active menace to the health of the population of the territory wherever his activities extend, and has without doubt done untold harm and very little good. . . .
>
> Yesterday I heard him advising a patient [who] had written in that he had a pain in his stomach at times, without relation to eating or the kind of food taken.
>
> His advice was to take milk and eggs for three weeks and if pain left him then this was a positive diagnosis of gastric or duodenal ulcer, and no matter where he went he could not get a more accurate diagnosis at the best hospital or clinic in the United States. . . .
>
> Perhaps this man might have an early malignancy. What then about the several weeks wasted? . . . Suppose this patient had a kidney involvement. What about all these eggs on such a condition?
>
> He prescribes and diagnoses cases without the least idea as to the person's condition; and if scientific equipment in the hands of men trained in its use is not more than 80 per cent efficient, how many times, I ask you, do you think this quack is right? . . .
>
> Ninety-five per cent of his correspondents are women. A great many of them are given very bad advice as to the care of the whole family, as any intelligent physician listening will tell you. As a competitor, he is not a competitor to me. I will reap a harvest from these people who are deferring visiting their physicians and having something corrected now which, if left alone, will lead to some surgical operation later on.

> But then it might be too late in many of these cases
> for surgery or anything else to do them any good.

Around the same time, Morris Fishbein received a letter from J. A. Garvin of Merck & Company. It seemed that Brinkley, for once at least, had thrown some trade their way:

> Dear Dr. Fishbein:
> . . . We have been recently startled by the unexplainable demand on the part of our customers for Sodium Borate C.P. Powder. From our representatives we have learned that a Dr. Brinkley, of Milford, Kansas, has broadcast recommendations for the use of Merck's Sodium Borate C.P. in obesity, and we have been literally swamped with orders, not only from the trade but also from the laity.
> We have taken action by notifying our . . . customers, as well as our sales staff and such retail druggists as have inquired of us regarding the product, strongly discouraging the use and sale of this material for the above mentioned purpose, as we are cognizant of the dangers involved in the internal administration of Sodium Borate.

Garvin asked if the AMA could take action. Fishbein passed the letter on to Arthur Cramp, who replied: "There is nothing the medical profession can do except to warn the public against the thing. Brinkley is getting to be a perfectly impossible problem. . . . His broadcasting is putrid!"

Putrid or not, the doctor's profits from *Medical Question Box* alone were now averaging $14,000 a week (or in today's currency, more than six and a half million dollars a year).

Fourteen thousand a week?

Corporate America was gobsmacked. Up till now the trafficker in barnyard testicles had been too outré, too down-market for the business world to acknowledge, but as news of *Medical Question Box* spread, and of the revenues it generated, things changed fast. Some executives were well advanced using radio ads themselves, despite the ossified thinking and church-lady interference they had to contend against. The crash of 1929 had made new approaches vital: something had to be done to *keep people buying.* Nevertheless, Brinkley hit some segments of the ad industry like a jolt of espresso: many realized for the first time that this "sordid pioneer of radio promotion," as Princeton's Dr. Young said, "had for six years been demonstrating how effective this method of advertising could be."

No more pussyfooting! American business seized the airwaves with a vengeance as every can, bottle, and box got its own song. The *Sunkist Musical Cocktail* program went toe-to-toe with Libby's Pineapple Picador and broadcasts from the Metropolitan Opera were interrupted by—what else?—Listerine: "Send those youngsters of yours into the bathroom for a good-night gargle." Everyone in commerce seemed to benefit except possibly Brinkley, for the great chatter of ads only further inflamed doctors against him, especially in the Midwest. With the AMA still banning advertising by its members, physicians were now among the lonely few not puffing their wares on the radio. Too many were peering into empty waiting rooms, their patients lost to *Medical Question Box.* In short, self-interest brought moral outrage to critical mass: doctors by the score appealed to Fishbein for help.

Something of a general without an army till now, Fishbein leapt at the opportunity. By now he saw plainly that the old strategy of containment—keeping Brinkley out of Chicago, out of California— would no longer suffice. The man had to be stopped cold. Proclaiming him "unquestionably the world's greatest charlatan," Fishbein vowed to bring every resource to bear—the AMA, the Federal Trade Commission, the Better Business Bureau, whatever it took—to put the

Milford Messiah out of action. He was a one-man national health emergency, Fishbein said, "treating dangerous afflictions by air." How many people had he harmed? None could say, but the anecdotal evidence was grave and growing. Given the vast size of his audience, carnage was statistically guaranteed.

Through reciprocity Brinkley had licenses to practice in several states. Fishbein traveled to each in turn, buttonholed the right people, and succeeded in having most of those permits yanked. He persuaded the London Medical Board to revoke Brinkley's right to practice in the United Kingdom. Enraged, Brinkley went on the radio to slam "Fishy Fishbein" and the other "smirking oligarchs" at the AMA. "These M.D.'s are a stinking, thieving, lying bunch," he said. "I'll grind their heads off under my heel like I would a snake."

As the charges flew back and forth, another well-known quack emerged as Brinkley's most conspicuous ally.

The business world may have been slow to catch on, but freer spirits had spotted Brinkley's brilliance almost from the get-go. Among those he inspired was Norman Baker, a long-jawed fire-eater from Iowa, who broke upon the scene with his inaugural broadcast over station KTNT on Thanksgiving Day 1925, and soon established himself as Brinkley's most successful disciple.

Baker had tasted fame already as a stage magician in vaudeville, flanked by a Madame Tangley, who read minds while levitating in midair, and an "electric man" he zapped nightly with "enough electricity to melt iron bars while held in ice water." After retiring like Prospero, Baker invented a portable calliope. He was teaching oil painting in ten lessons by mail when one night his radio dial found KFKB.

On a bluff overlooking the Mississippi River, Baker founded a station of his own. Promising meek Muscatine, Iowa, that he would lift it "from being a little burg lost in the cornfields to a city the whole world knows about," he set about doing it on the Brinkley model, sans goats. Over KTNT ("Know the Naked Truth") he flogged rank patent medicines, interspersing his spiels with "honest to goodness" radio for plain folk, down-home tunes, and the comedy duo of Daffy and Gloomy. Unlike Brinkley, Norman Baker liked to bellow. Otherwise, for a man who wore purple shirts and purple ties, drove a purple car, and wrote with lavender ink, he was strikingly unoriginal. In fact he would follow Brinkley's lead so slavishly over the next fifteen years that he became a sort of violet shadow trailing him from place to place, aping his career moves point for point, in a long, vain attempt to beat the master at his own game.

For now though, in the 1929 uproar over *Medical Question Box,* he joined forces with Brinkley and launched his own robust attacks on the AMA. True, this was less to help a brother quack than to protect his own franchise, which was just taking off. For after dabbling in remedies of his own—curing appendicitis with onions was one— Baker had stumbled on his destiny just months earlier when he broke into cancer cures. His first was a paste used to remove leg knots from horses, but in December he announced a new drinkable treatment created in collaboration with Dr. Charles Ozias of Kansas City, distinguished member of the American Association for Medico-Physical Research and Defensive Diet League of America. The ingredients were a trade secret.

One glassful did the job.

Baker opened his cancer-curing refreshment stand at his new hospital in Muscatine, a converted roller rink. In came the patients; out (rumor had it) went the bodies and the suitcases full of cash.

New Year's Eve 1929. Beverly Hills, California.

Dr. Morris Fishbein and his wife, Anna, rang in the new decade at the block-long hacienda of screenwriter Herman Mankiewicz. A poker player with the Schlogl's crowd on his trips through Chicago, Mankiewicz had lured Fishbein's old chum Ben Hecht out here to write for the movies with one immortal telegram: "Millions are to be grabbed out here and your only competition is idiots." At the party that night was the cream of moviedom: Charlie Chaplin, Gary Cooper, Janet Gaynor. Another star, Kay Francis, walked over to Fishbein, introduced herself, and sat in his lap. Lacing her fingers around his neck, Miss Francis made experiments with her rear end until she was comfortable.

"Tell me frankly," she said, "am I the best-dressed woman in Hollywood?"

26

At the start of 1930 *Radio Digest* announced that Brinkley's KFKB was the most popular radio station in the United States. In a national survey it had received more than four times as many votes as the second-place finisher and thirty-five times more than KFKB's local rival, WDAF, owned by the *Kansas City Star*.

Simultaneously, Fishbein crowned Brinkley "the most daring and the most dangerous" charlatan in the country—out of 125,000 on file—and vowed again in the April issue of *JAMA* to have him, and Norman Baker, too, taken off the air for good: "The Federal Radio Commission must be depended upon [to end] the obscene mouthing and pernicious promotions that are broadcast by the stations that these quacks dominate."

Brinkley thanked him for the attack. "This scrap on us has caused the people to come to us in such increased numbers we're swamped completely," he told his listeners. But the threat to his station was real, and he knew it. He stepped up his mailings.

> My dear radio Friend:
>
> Thousands of letters and affidavits have arrived pledging me your support in the present hour of trial. I appreciate your loyalty more than you will ever know. . . .
>
> Now don't sit back and think your job is done. . . . Appoint yourself a committee of ONE to see the listeners of KFKB, have them wire or write the Federal

Radio Commission at Washington, D.C., and tell the
TRUTH about me and my policies. Have your friends
to see their friends and have letters written and wires
sent. . . .

After our honor has been vindicated may the God of
Peace continue to watch over and keep us.

The battle, he thought, was well in hand. Then he learned that
Fishbein was also trying to have his Kansas medical license revoked.
Brinkley lost his temper like a noon whistle and ran a full-page ad
syndicated in several newspapers:

I DEFY THE AMERICAN MEDICAL ASSOCIATION!

But then he calmed down. When the *Kansas City Star,* in unoffi-
cial league with Fishbein, launched a scorching series of exposés
about his storied career, Brinkley even granted the paper an interview.
"Do I look like I am worrying? I am not worrying," he told reporter
A. B. McDonald. "The American Medical Association has been fighting me for ten years and I have licked them every time."

With a race for Kansas governor looming, Brinkley could afford
to sound smug. None of the candidates and few of their backers
wanted to tangle with a figure so many voters adored. Indeed the
Topeka Daily State Journal found that Fishbein's attacks on the goat-
gland man had produced quite a "showing of perspiration in political
circles," and the odds were now that "while some gestures may be
made toward Doctor Brinkley, he really won't be hit with anything
except well padded gloves." Just look at all his important friends.
"While William A. Smith, attorney general, is taking the lead in the
gathering of evidence with which to try to revoke the doctor's [med-
ical] license, Percy S. Walker, Smith's brother-in-law, is head of the
Brinkley Association of Druggists," the *Kansas City Journal-Post*
reminded readers. "Col. James E. Smith, son-in-law of Governor
[Clyde] Reed, is one of the attorneys for Dr. Brinkley." To say nothing

of Charles Curtis, the Kansan who was now vice president of the United States; Governor Reed himself; and James G. Strong, the congressman from Brinkley's district, all of whom he had cultivated like prize vegetables.

A few days later the *Journal-Post* ran a multipage mash note to Brinkley, a paid promotional spread disguised as news. It was filled with photographs of his extended family: entertainers, nurses, mail-room girls, the gardener. There was the legendary Bill Stittsworth in his battered hat. And who was that, Happy Harry? One look at that face, and it was as if you'd known him all your life.

27

It was a little after midnight. Norman Baker and his chief aide, Harry Hoxsey, sat in Baker's office at KTNT, unwinding with a couple of whiskies. Through the picture window they had a royal view of the Mississippi River, all glints and shadows at this hour. A lighted barge went sliding by. Life was good. Applications for space at the cancer clinic had reached three hundred a day.

But success had its price: the KTNT compound had acquired the atmosphere of an armed camp. Just a few days earlier Fishbein had called Baker "a ghoul," and thanks in part to such rhetoric, Baker and most of his employees carried guns now. It was a publicity stunt only up to a point. Teased about his revolver, a staff doctor said sharply that he kept it handy because the AMA "was after him."

The telephone on Baker's desk rang. Hoxsey put down his drink and answered.

"Mr. Baker had better not come down," said a muffled voice. "There are three tough-looking guys parked across the street in an old Buick." Hoxsey told his boss and the two went pounding downstairs to investigate, just in time to spot three men running low behind a hedge. The pair ducked back inside and doused the lights as the first shots blistered the doorframe. Hoxsey, who had grabbed a gun on his way down, fired back. The shots echoing across the compound roused voices in nearby buildings, then cries and confusion. Hoxsey was firing blindly as Baker ran upstairs for his own pistol. Suddenly there was a yell of pain from the bushes.

Two shadows emerged, bent low, dragging a third toward their car. They shoved the injured man inside, jumped in after him, and sped away.

Next day the Associated Press headlined the story:

GUN FIGHT CLIMAXES FIGHT WITH DR. FISHBEIN

Police found streaks of blood on the grass but no other clues. The gunmen were assumed to be AMA sympathizers. Hirelings perhaps? Baker rode that theory hard, even claiming that Fishbein himself— "the Jewish dominator of the medical trust in America"—had been one of the shooters. The editor was able to prove, however, that he was in Chicago's Presbyterian Hospital on the night in question having an operation for hemorrhoids. Despite the police report, *JAMA* claimed to doubt that this "lurid incident" had even taken place.

The drive to revoke Brinkley's medical license was gathering steam. Not fast enough for some: Dr. John F. Hassig, head of the state medical board, complained to a colleague that the effort was "up against the strongest political combination that could possibly have been assembled by any one person." After visiting Attorney General William Smith three times urging him to pursue the case, Hassig had to force him to action with threats. Finally on April 29 the Kansas State Medical Board, backed by the AMA, filed formal charges against the doctor for "gross immorality and unprofessional conduct." This was catnip to the *Kansas City Star*, whose semiprincipled campaign against "the goat-gland quack" had been running for weeks. (A local commentator listed three motives behind the *Star*'s vendetta: "[I]t could build up a big reader-interest by making a sensational exposé of the Brinkley operations; it could crush Brinkley and kill off the competition which his radio station offered to its station; it could win the undying gratitude of all the ethical doctors in every town and village throughout the land.")

Combing the Midwest for Brinkley victims, the *Star*'s top newshound reported an embarrassment of riches. "I have gone into homes and found men bedridden, ruined by the bungling butchery of this man Brinkley," A. B. McDonald wrote. "I have found women crippled for life, crouching in wheel chairs. I have found men who went to Brinkley . . . and now they are like Lazarus who lay at the gate covered with sores."

Some stories of his "merciless cupidity" went back more than ten years. Mrs. Cora Maddox described how as a fifteen-year-old appendicitis patient she had been held prisoner by the doctor ("using the vilest language I ever heard") while he demanded an extra hundred dollars for the operation he had just performed: "I lay at the point of death while [Brinkley, drunk] straddled the doorway with a revolver in his hand and threatened to shoot my two brothers if they did not pay him." McDonald also unearthed disaffected ex-employees. Mrs. Ferris, a nurse, called her former boss "diabolical. . . . He is the most cruel, pitiless, cold-blooded man I have ever known." Grace Jenkins said she had quit her job after just twenty-four hours: "I helped nurse a very rich publisher from London, who had paid Dr. Brinkley $2,000 for the goat gland operation, and he was in a desperate condition with blood poison and a sloughing wound. I saw an old man brought in who was paralyzed and he paid Dr. Brinkley $750 for the goat gland operation upon Brinkley's assurance that it would cure him of his paralysis.

"It was too much for me. I would not have stayed there if he had paid me $1,000 a day."

But the *Star*'s most sensational charge was that Brinkley had killed some of his patients.

He denied it. "I will not accept any patient who cannot be cured or who may die under treatment," he said. "No patient of mine has ever died here. If we should have a man die here the doctors who are fighting me would publish it all over the country, so I must be careful. Other doctors may kill 'em off, but I daren't."

The next day the *Star* published the names of five people who had expired at Brinkley's hospital since the fall of 1928. His signature was on their death certificates.

More names—many more—would follow.

28

Minnie was frightened by the ferocity of the attacks, but Brinkley just laughed. "Darling, I've learned a lot from goats," he said. "Did you ever see a billy butt?"

That she had. For years her husband had been sending a goon squad of Pinkerton detectives, who moonlighted as his security guards, to drop in on obstreperously dissatisfied former patients. The same crew had called on some of the doctors in nearby Junction City to suggest they stop bad-mouthing Dr. Brinkley to people who were changing trains. These muscle-bound emissaries didn't hurt anybody. They didn't have to. One of them, Howard Hale Wilson—someone described him as a "male secretary and fixer . . . with hands like hams"—explained that "if anybody ever gets in the way of my boss I'll fix him like this," and mimed throttling.

Now as state investigators followed up the *Star*'s interviews with victims, some of them suddenly and mysteriously didn't remember complaining. It turned out the doctor had switched to carrots this time and was offering to pay well for signed retractions.

Sometimes he got them. A Kansas farmer named S. A. Hittle had publicly reviled Brinkley for having "ruined" him and was threatening to sue. But after henchmen with a checkbook drove from Milford to visit, he signed an affidavit retracting his complaints. His family insisted on the truth of his original claim, and two doctors who had seen him postop agreed. "When Mr. Hittle came to me," said Dr. John G. Sheldon of Kansas City, "I found an infected bladder attached to the skin, draining to the outside through the abdomen and a large stone imbedded in the neck of the bladder. . . . The wound at that time was not healed and is not healed yet." Dr. R. E. Eagen of Springhill, who had warned Hittle not to go to Milford in the first place, described it as "a nasty, dirty wound in his abdomen inflicted by Brinkley and filled with running pus. . . . You may state for me that Dr. Brinkley butchered Mr. Hittle and it was a dirty job of butchering at that." Maybe so, but he was off the witness list.

Meanwhile Brinkley hired detectives to dig up dirt on every member of the Kansas medical board who would decide his fate—if things ever got that far. In a battle that swiftly reached the U.S. Supreme Court, Brinkley's attorneys argued that the whole proceeding should be quashed because the medical board, being outside the legal system, had no power to judge or to punish. As for the issue of diagnosing patients over the radio, his team produced a statement by Dr. Morris Fishbein "in which Fishbein asserted that television later would come into general medical use and the doctors would not see patients directly, but would prescribe for them after looking at the television pictures." It followed therefore that with *Medical Question Box,* "the Milford doctor was just a step ahead of Dr. Fishbein."

From May 5 to 8, 1930, the Kansas Medical Society held its annual convention at the Jayhawk Hotel in Topeka. Cleaning up the profession—that is, getting rid of Brinkley—was Topic A. There to rally the brethren was keynote speaker Dr. Morris Fishbein.

With his quick bark, à la Walter Winchell, he was "a regular machine gun of oratory, shooting his short, snappy sentences with a swiftness difficult to follow." But nobody that night missed his meaning. Fishbein savaged Brinkley without mentioning his name by limning the quintessential charlatan, "a man who is likely to have a pleasing personality, a smooth tongue, able to present his case with eloquence. He will claim educational advantages he does not possess. He will display a large number of diplomas, usually from questionable or foreign schools, and always he will produce a large number of testimonials from the professional testimonial givers." Cheers and laughter filled the smoky hall.

Next day as the editor strode through the lobby, a Shawnee County sheriff's deputy slapped a summons against his chest. Brinkley was suing him for defamation. As word ran through the hotel, his fellow M.D.'s were outraged, but Fishbein shrugged it off. "It is quite the common thing for persons exposed by the American Medical Association to file suit," he said. He then upped the ante by insulting Brinkley even more bluntly, calling him "a menace to humanity" whose "quackery and butchery" had often required lifesaving heroics by real doctors. Sue away, Fishbein said. "The standing head in the *Journal* is and will continue to be: 'John R. Brinkley, Quack.'"

The editor coolly predicted that the suit would never go to trial, and he turned out to be right. After squeezing some righteous publicity from it, Brinkley eventually let it drop on a technicality. He had other things to worry about.

The Supreme Court had ruled against him. This meant that right after the FRC hearing on his radio license, now almost upon him, he would have to confront the Kansas medical board to fight for his other license, too. In this hour of need he appealed to cancer quack Norman Baker to help him map strategy in their common fight against Washington and the "giant octopus" of the AMA.

Sometime back the Iowan had bought fifteen hundred dollars' worth of radio equipment from Brinkley and never paid the bill. But caught in the pincers of the Federal Radio Commission and the state medical board, the doctor wasn't holding a grudge. He wrote pressing the need for a united front, reminding Baker that "KTNT is to be taken off the air as well as KFKB, providing the American Medical Association can do it. . . . I presume if I lose they will fight you and if I win they won't cite you. Therefore, it would seem that any help you can throw my way would be helping yourself." In solidarity Brinkley enclosed some tips on "affidavit-gathering techniques."

Baker ignored him. Instead on May 12, 1930, he hosted a thrill-packed festival in Muscatine with more than thirty thousand true believers. "Cancer is conquered!" Baker boomed, bestriding the narrow stage in eye-popping purple as a sea of hands groped the air and hosannas rose from the multitude. Vaudeville acts followed, and testimonials; then Baker himself reappeared holding aloft—what was it? A vial of the precious elixir! Magic in a glass! Enough medicine, he thundered, to rid not one, not two, but *twenty-five patients* of the last particle of cancer. He showed the tumbler here, there, raised it high, then drank it off with a flourish—proof positive it was as safe as it was effective.

For the grand finale a sixty-eight-year-old farmer named Mandus Johnson was led to a chair on the stage. Very slowly the long bandage on his head was unwound. A Baker staff surgeon peeled back his scalp . . . then part of his skull. . . . Johnson lowered his head, and what looked like cancerous brain matter was exposed to the audience. The brain was then salted with a "special powder" created by Baker and the scalp replaced. The farmer stood and shook hands with the surgeon.

Some fainted; some threw up; most cheered like mad.

29

In its short life the Federal Radio Commission (ancestor of the Federal Communications Commission) had been so busy riding the whirlwind of broadcasting that real regulation had barely begun. It took Morris Fishbein's relentless pestering to get it to move on Brinkley. Well aware of this, and nursing resentment the size of an oil reserve, the doctor nonetheless decided to treat his summons to Washington like an invitation to the president's ball. He offered to pay for a whole trainload of fans to come with him and enjoy the fun. Told the price, he changed his mind, but thirty-five supporters still bought tickets themselves. What a time of year to visit the capital! Along the Potomac the cherry trees were laden with pink popcorn, and ranks of tulips guarded the White House. The morning of the hearing the whole group chattered expectantly behind the doctor— two or three holding goat-gland babies—as he entered the august chamber at the Department of the Interior to take on the FRC.

But the fun was over. "The commission is not satisfied that this station is operated for the public interest," intoned chairman Ira Robinson, a man who looked and sounded like a stranger to happy endings, as he and his four fellow commissioners stared down on opposing counsel: for the assorted complainants, W. C. Ralston, assistant attorney general of Kansas; for the defense, George E. Strong, son of the U.S. congressman who was Brinkley's longtime chum. Farther back, in the horseshoe of seats allotted to the public, Arthur Cramp had slipped in unobserved.

Mrs. Bertha Lacey, one of the doctor's most loyal "lady fans," testified first. In the patient style of a kindergarten teacher she explained to the commission how *Medical Question Box* worked: "You just listen over the radio to what the other ladies [write] about their symptoms, and you'd be awful dumb if you didn't know what was the matter with you." Until Compound No. 150 came into her life, she herself had been a martyr to constipation; now she had all ten members of her family on it. "It is not only good," she said, "it is wonderful."

In all about thirty of Brinkley's admirers took the stand, including members of his radio staff. Some may have helped him less than they hoped, as when *MQB* secretary Ruth Athey mentioned his knack for prescribing "the proper remedies at a glance." And Commissioner Robinson, hitching forward on his elbows, roughly interrupted along the way, pressing witnesses to cut to the chase: "Is this radio station a mere adjunct of Brinkley's practice and hospital? Is he using it simply to make money? Why do his prescriptions cost so much more than usual?" The commissioner owned a farm in West Virginia, he said; he doubted he could get a radio license to advertise his livestock.

Minnie Brinkley jumped up. "Can I say a few words?" she cried before friendly hands tugged her back into her chair.

On the advice of his attorneys the doctor didn't testify himself, lest the Kansas medical board try to turn his own words against him. But after hearing his supporters for a day and a half, backed by two hundred affidavits from patients back home, the panel looked not only unimpressed but increasingly sullen—brightening only for opposing testimony like that of Dr. Hugh Young of Johns Hopkins University, who called *Medical Question Box* "the greatest possible danger" to the public health. Among the affidavits attacking Brinkley was one from Dr. Gilley back in Kansas, who detailed how the medicine prescribed over KFKB had killed Edward Humrickhouse, mail carrier.

W. C. Ralston was just rising to make his closing statement when

Brinkley broke in. Did the commission object to *Medical Question Box*? Very well. He would cancel the program.

Making so many people goggle at once must have given the imp in Brinkley some pleasure. Sacrificing his cash cow did not, but it was plain to him which way the wind was blowing, and he figured it was better to cut his losses and keep his station. As he liked to boast, he could "think of three ways to get rich before breakfast." There was plenty more where *MQB* came from.

And that was that—or it should have been. The chief mandate of the FRC had been to decide whether Brinkley had exceeded the bounds of normal advertising in his use of the public airwaves; remove *MQB,* and the question was moot. But there was a niggling charge still undisposed of. Bluenoses in the field had been reporting back to Washington that his radio talks were "obscene and extremely disgusting." Words most people handled with tongs, like *erection* and *climax,* he employed as a matter of course, to say nothing of his light-hearted take on the Sixth Commandment: "I suggest you have your husband sterilized, and then you will be safe, providing you don't get out in anybody else's cow pasture and get in with some other bull." Talk like that might tickle the yokels, but it scandalized the professional offense takers monitoring him on hotel-room radios.

Giving up *Medical Question Box* worked, almost. On June 13 his license to broadcast was canceled by a vote of 3 to 2. "Station KFKB is conducted only in the personal interest of Dr. John R. Brinkley," declared Commissioner Robinson in announcing the majority's ruling, but the talk on the street was that the doc had been sandbagged by the puritans.

He didn't chop up a car this time, but he was plenty mad. Still broadcasting pending appeal, Brinkley accused President Hoover and the AMA of a criminal conspiracy to fix the verdict: "I am informed by a friend whose name I am not at liberty to disclose that the American Medical Association spent [either $15,000 or $50,000, reception unclear] with those three members of the Federal Radio

Commission, the money being paid to them through one of the attorneys of the Federal Radio Commission." Then suddenly his tone changed.

"If you people think that myself and my station have been crucified and will tell your congressmen and senators, I may get my radio license back. . . . Now I shall discuss some of the beatitudes of Jesus as they came from His mouth on the Mount of Olives."

"Build Up Personality, Magnetism, Vitality with Violet Rays!" Electricity could make you more interesting. *From* Medicine: Perspectives in History and Art, *courtesy of Bob Greenspan, M.D.*

Fashionable as the newest form of capital punishment, electricity was also touted as the cure for almost any ailment. In 1913 John Brinkley claimed to be an "electro medic." *From* Medicine: Perspectives in History and Art, *courtesy of Bob Greenspan, M.D.*

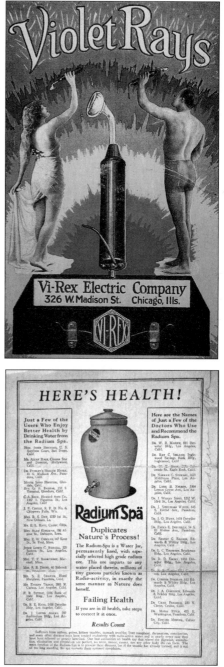

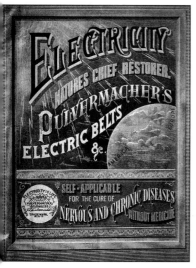

Radium-laced water was a popular, up-to-date health drink until 1932, when industrialist Eben Byers, a three-bottle-a-day man, died hideously from the accumulated poison. The *Wall Street Journal* headlined the story: "The Radium Water Worked Fine Until His Jaw Came Off." *From* Medicine: Perspectives in History and Art, *courtesy of Bob Greenspan, M.D.*

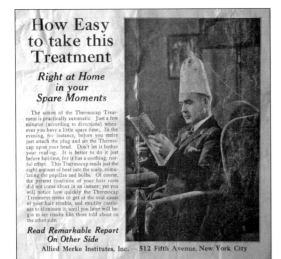

How Easy to take this Treatment

Right at Home in your Spare Moments

The action of the Thermocap Treatment is practically automatic. Just a few minutes (according to directions) whenever you have a little spare time. In the evening, for instance, before you retire just attach the plug and set the Thermocap upon your head. Don't let it bother your reading. It is better to do it just before bedtime, for it has a soothing, restful effect. This Thermocap sends just the right amount of heat into the scalp, stimulating the papillae and bulbs. Of course, the present condition of your hair roots did not come about in an instant; yet you will notice how quickly the Thermocap Treatment seems to get at the real cause of your hair trouble, and steadily continues to eliminate it, until you later will begin to see results like those told about on the other side.

Read Remarkable Report On Other Side

Allied Merke Institutes, Inc. — 512 Fifth Avenue, New York City

This electric fez claimed to grow hair, thanks to "blue light from a special actinic quartz ray bulb." *From Medicine: Perspectives in History and Art, courtesy of Bob Greenspan, M.D.*

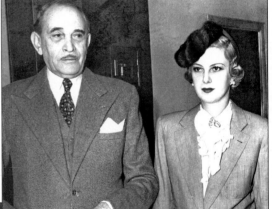

Dr. Serge Voronoff and his third wife, Gertrude, aka the Condesa da Foz. Voronoff contended that installing monkey glands in people could make them live for a hundred fifty years. *AP Images*

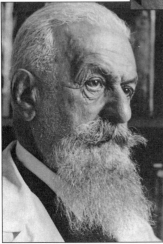

Dr. Eugen Steinach, Voronoff's Viennese rival. He believed lost youth could be restored with vasectomies and ovarian radiation. *AP Images*

Before he became the great quackbuster of his day, Morris Fishbein of the American Medical Association had a brief career as a practicing physician. *Courtesy of Michael Marks and the Fishbein family*

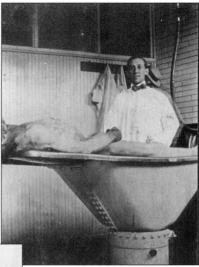

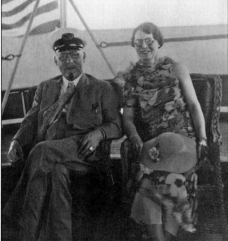

The wealthiest quack of the age, Dr. John Brinkley cruised aboard his yacht each summer with his wife, Minnie. He was a champion deep-sea fisherman. *Whitehead Memorial Museum*

Bring on the goat: Brinkley and his wife in surgery at their famous Milford, Kansas, clinic. *Kansas State Historical Society*

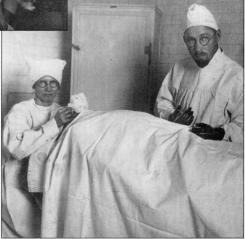

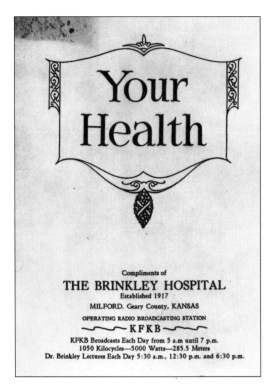

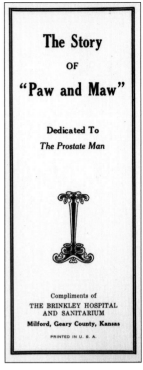

Brinkley was a pioneer of modern advertising, both by mail and over the radio. *Kansas State Historical Society*

Parable of the prostate: So miraculous was his treatment, Brinkley said, it would make his name "stand out in bold relief among the great luminaries of this generation." *Kansas State Historical Society*

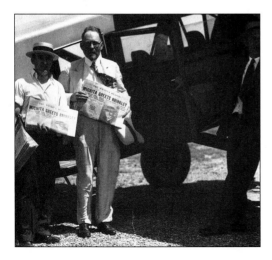

Gubernatorial candidate Brinkley *(right)* with unidentified henchman, probably 1930. The doctor's use of an airplane would revolutionize American political campaigning. *Kansas State Historical Society*

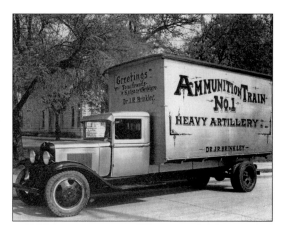

The centerpiece of Brinkley's cavalcade in his run for Kansas governor in 1932. The back opened out into a stage for speeches and music. *Kansas State Historical Society*

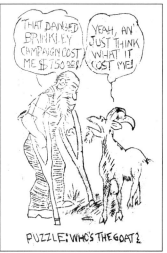

The crutches are significant here: over the years many patients left Brinkley's clinic crippled or dead. *Kansas State Historical Society*

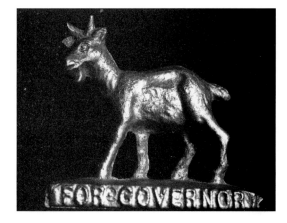

An empire built on goat glands launched Brinkley toward the Kansas governorship. *Kansas State Historical Society*

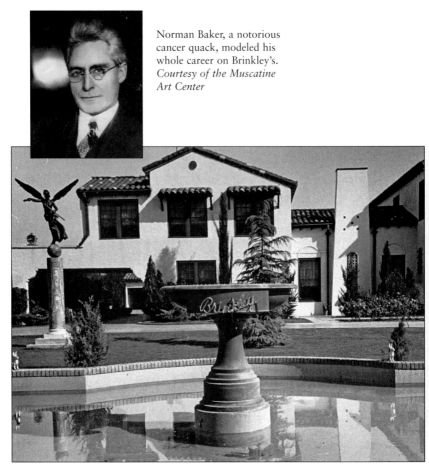

Norman Baker, a notorious cancer quack, modeled his whole career on Brinkley's. *Courtesy of the Muscatine Art Center*

Brinkley's mansion in Del Rio, Texas, near the Rio Grande. He enlivened the estate with Galápagos tortoises, penguins, and monkeys. *Getty Images*

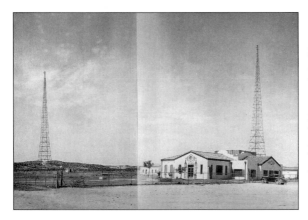

In Mexico, out of the reach of American authorities, Brinkley built his "border blaster," XERA. At a million watts, it was the most powerful radio station in the world. *Whitehead Memorial Museum*

Along with his shameless quackery, Brinkley broadcast great country music. The legendary Carter Family became national stars performing on XERA. *Back row, left to right:* A.P., Janette, unidentified announcer, Sara, and Maybelle. *Front row:* Helen, Anita, and June. *Carter Family Museum*

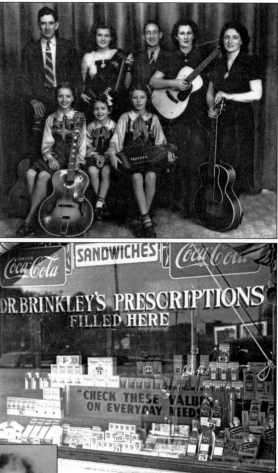

By creating the Brinkley Pharmaceutical Association, the doctor found yet another way to make money. A vast network of druggists sold his "cures" for about six times retail. *Getty Images*

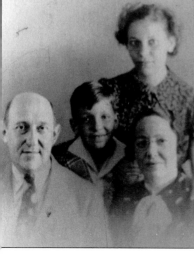

In 1937 the Fishbein family had a fateful encounter with the Brinkleys on board a luxury liner. *Clockwise from left:* Morris, son Justin, daughter Marjorie, and wife Anna. *Courtesy of Michael Marks and the Fishbein family*

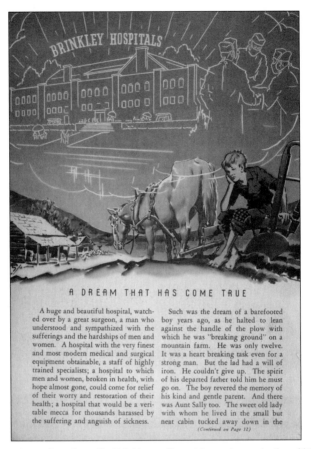

A DREAM THAT HAS COME TRUE

A huge and beautiful hospital, watched over by a great surgeon, a man who understood and sympathized with the sufferings and the hardships of men and women. A hospital with the very finest and most modern medical and surgical equipment obtainable, a staff of highly trained specialists; a hospital to which men and women, broken in health, with hope almost gone, could come for relief of their worry and restoration of their health; a hospital that would be a veritable mecca for thousands harassed by the suffering and anguish of sickness.

Such was the dream of a barefooted boy years ago, as he halted to lean against the handle of the plow with which he was "breaking ground" on a mountain farm. He was only twelve. It was a heart breaking task even for a strong man. But the lad had a will of iron. He couldn't give up. The spirit of his departed father told him he must go on. The boy revered the memory of his kind and gentle parent. And there was Aunt Sally too. The sweet old lady with whom he lived in the small but neat cabin tucked away down in the

(Continued on Page 12)

In print and on the radio Brinkley wallowed in sentimental tales of his childhood—a savvy commercial ploy. *Kansas State Historical Society*

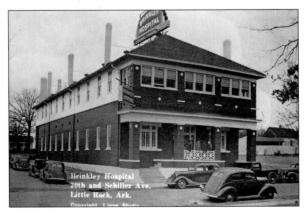

Brinkley built his third and last hospital in Little Rock, Arkansas. He later came to regret it. *Kansas State Historical Society*

30

Six weeks later—on July 15, 1930—the Kansas Board of Medical Examiners met to consider revoking the doctor's other license.

Outside the Kansan Hotel in Topeka, goat-gland recipients were cutting capers and doing handstands for the press. It wasn't yet nine A.M. and the sun was already baking the plaza, but when Brinkley arrived, he stepped from his Cadillac collared, buttoned, and bejeweled: diamond tiepin, diamond-studded tie clasp, diamond studs, and two diamond rings, one with a gem the size of a human eye. There was a queasy excitement in the air, for no one was quite sure what he was walking into, including the doctor himself. In Wisconsin farmer Henry Dorn was facing his state medical board on charges of sorcery.

Inside seventy-five people packed the hearing room. But if they had been brought there, as a pro-Brinkley paper complained, by "the fanatical fervor of a certain official of the A.M.A.," that official was not among them. Fearing his presence might rouse the rabble to demonstrations or worse, Fishbein was keeping out of sight. He wanted the hearing to look like community theater, not an auto-da-fé arranged by outsiders. Backstage, however, he was full of advice.

"Rotten grafter!"

"Dirty crook!"

The first session had barely begun when "a spirited exchange of personalities" broke out between Brinkley attorney Fred Jackson and reporter A. B. McDonald of the *Star*. Three or four men clamped Jackson in his chair as he struggled to launch himself on the newsman.

Order was restored, but it was a fair barometer of the tension in the room, exacerbated as time passed by oxygen deprivation. By noon the hottest summer Kansas had ever known had turned the hearing room into hell in a box.

Brinkley alone kept his suit coat on. During opening arguments he sat at the defense table smoking perfumed cigarettes with the élan of a patron at an outdoor café. Seated behind him and staring balefully at the back of his head was mangled ex-patient John Zahner.

Another former patient, R. J. Hibbard, was first up for the prosecution. His slow shuffle toward the witness stand as he groped the air spoke volumes. His wife, who testified next, said that on his return home after getting his goat glands, Mr. Hibbard had lain in bed unconscious for three days.

More of the mauled and mutilated followed. Charles Ziegenharth, sixty, said that instead of stitching him up properly after a prostate operation, Brinkley had plugged the bleeding wound with a piece of rubber boot heel and sent him on his way. Grant Eden, caretaker of a state park, had come in on the same bus as John Zahner. He, too, got "the works," after which he could barely move. When he later wrote to complain, Brinkley replied with a note describing the hunting trip he had just returned from, ending with: "Your condition is your own fault. . . . Wishing you a merry Christmas." There was testimony from Robert Carroll, brother of Cora Maddox, whose vivid account of Brinkley's gunplay at the clinic had already run in the *Star*. "I smelled whiskey on his breath," Carroll said. "He opened a desk drawer, took out a revolver and told me my sister would not come out of that hospital except over his dead body, unless he was paid $100 more." Carroll and his brother had returned with guns of their own and rescued her Wild West–style from the building.

By the third day of testimony, July 17, one medical-board member was so incensed that he interrupted the hearing to demand an immediate verdict of guilty. After Brinkley's rights were reexplained to the panelist, John Zahner took the stand.

His tale of woe mirrored others at first: how the operation at the

Milford clinic (he was reluctant to admit it was for goat glands) had left him broken in body and spirit. A day or so after the procedure, he said, when the pain was worse than ever, he confronted the "little man with funny whiskers" in the hall:

"Doctor, I am five times as bad as when I came."

"That's natural and to be expected; it will be a year before you are fully well."

"But they told me I would be well in three days. Your wife told me that."

"You must have misunderstood her. You may have to come back for another operation later on."

Zahner had returned home to Lenexa, where he took to his bed and lost weight. Consumed with his own suffering, he failed to notice at first the new wallpaper and better lamps in the house. Nor did he register his wife Minerva's rising impatience as the days passed without his crossing the river Styx. After two weeks she could bear it no longer. "I'm leaving you," she said. Zahner, in no shape to argue, gave her two thousand dollars and arranged for one of his hired men, Pat McDougan, to drive her back to her family in Indiana.

Quite possibly Minerva and McDougan were already having an affair: she had once interceded to keep him from being fired. Now as they set out on their trip, McDougan warned her that it was dangerous for a woman to be carrying two thousand dollars in cash, so she gave him fourteen hundred of it to keep for her. In Kansas City they rented a motel room, and during the night he disappeared with the car.

Minerva returned home with her nosegay of disappointments and one purpose, to make her husband's life a living hell. She even trailed him into the hearing room. After Zahner hauled himself from the witness stand, she offered an affidavit to the board contending that he "returned from the Brinkley institution and did not take care of himself, that he went out in the rain and did heavy physical labor which ruined any benefits he might have obtained."

The rest of the prosecution's case consisted of expert witnesses with withering opinions of Brinkley's work. Dr. Thomas G. Orr of the

University of Kansas School of Medicine said the goat-gland graft Brinkley claimed to perform was "absolutely impossible," a professor of urology called the procedure "so silly it is ridiculous," and a third said it would have no effect at all "unless he introduced infection with it," as he frequently managed to do. One testified as an eyewitness. Dr. R. R. Cave of Manhattan, Kansas, had journeyed to Brinkley's clinic the year before out of simple curiosity. Cave had already studied Brinkley's illustrated pamphlet outlining the four-phase compound operation—how he transplanted "an artery and a nerve so as to increase the blood and nerve supply to certain organs . . . to strengthen them and rejuvenate them"; how he shrank enlarged prostates by cutting off the blood supply. But when Cave viewed the procedures for himself, he was surprised to find that "no attempt was made to do any of these things," that the doctor just put "little pellets" in the patient's scrotum and sewed him up. "This particular patient," Dr. Cave added, "complained bitterly of pain throughout the operation. . . . Brinkley insisted he was 'mistaken.'"

Cross-examining these experts, Brinkley's lawyers could do little but insult them and be insulted in return:

Q: I wouldn't pay you money for advice at any time.
A: Well, I might have the same opinion of you as a lawyer.

The defense was looking at long odds when it opened its case on July 22.

Rebuttal of the charges began, as expected, with a volley of testimonials. Leonidas F. Richardson of York, Nebraska, raved about the miracles his goat glands had achieved in curing his diabetes, kidney, and prostate problems "almost in the twinkling of an eye." Next, a rejuvenated sixty-eight-year-old offered to jump over a table. A few of these happy customers weren't sure if they'd received goat glands or not—"but I shouldn't wonder," said one, "for I've been wanting to chew sprouts." On they came, a bank president, a doctor, oil speculators, clerks, a full forty of them before the medical board called a halt.

Then Dr. Brinkley himself took the stand. Outside, Topeka gasped in 103-degree heat. Inside it was little better, yet he still wore his coat.

"You'll be more comfortable if you take it off," his attorney said.

The doctor glanced over at the prosecution table and laughed good-naturedly. "Maybe I'll be a little hotter later on," he said. "I'd better keep it on till then." The smile disappeared. "I am here to defend myself against unrighteous attacks on my professional integrity and ability," he said. "The issues are even broader than this.... [T]hey involve the right of physicians to adopt and use new methods, even if they have not been approved by those in control of the American Medical Association."

Steered by attorney Fred Jackson, Brinkley spent the afternoon refuting specific charges one by one. Regarding his much-quoted claim that no patient had ever died in his hospital: "I did not mean to say that. What I meant to say was that no patient had ever died in my hospital from a compound operation, and I believe that no person ever died from that operation after he left my hospital. . . . There is no danger connected with it." All the allegations against him sprang from malice or ignorance, he said. He was not a sot. He had never been struck on the head with a board. As to claims that Dr. Max Thorek, with whom he had once studied, regarded him as a charlatan: "Dr. Thorek is a very lovely gentleman," he said, "and he and I are the warmest personal friends." After a couple of mild jokes and a genial reference to "this little show we're putting on here," Brinkley's direct testimony came to a close at five P.M.

When he took the stand next morning for cross-examination, he wasn't wearing his coat.

For several hours prosecutor William Smith tried to crack Brinkley's studied aplomb. He couldn't do it. But as it turned out, he didn't need to. Sometimes ignorance has an eloquence of its own:

Q: You say in the literature you furnish a new blood supply and you furnish new nerve supply to the testicle?

A: Yes sir.
Q: How do they benefit the testicle?
A: Well I believe they do; that is my opinion.
Q: How?
A: I can't explain it.
Q: Is it in any textbook?
A: I don't know.
Q: Did you learn it in school?
A: I don't know that I did.
Q: How do you know it?
A: From the results I get with my patients.

Brinkley reaffirmed that this surgery held "no danger"—whereupon Smith snatched up a fistful of documents and held them high. They were death certificates signed by Brinkley, all belonging to patients who had succumbed at his clinic—men and women, young and old. Forty-two people, some of whom weren't ill when they arrived, had died either by his own hand or under his supervision. Six at least were victims of goat-gland operations gone awry. The others were variously dead of nephritis, peritonitis, appendicitis, "syptic thrombus," and gangrene. If in 1930 that didn't make Brinkley a murderer in the eyes of the law—and it didn't—well, wasn't that a scandal in itself? The man was running a corpse factory.

He tried to save himself then, much as he had in Washington, with a daring late-inning play. He invited the board to visit Milford to see a goat-gland operation for themselves. Fairness demanded it, he said. With great reluctance the panel members agreed to make the trip.

They came. They saw.

Two days later, Brinkley's license was revoked.

31

A lesser man might have crawled off whimpering into the shadows. Brinkley's response was to run for governor.

He announced his candidacy in Wichita on September 20, three days after losing his medical license. "Thousands of Kansans have written urging me to run for governor," he said. "Judging from my mail the people of Kansas seem to believe that I have been persecuted, not prosecuted, and as long as I have a leg to stand on I will fight." He promised the public not to wage a "campaign of vindictiveness," except in one forgivable regard. "You will perhaps recall . . . that I filed a suit against the American Medical Association and its secretary, Morris Fishbein, several months ago. . . . Since that time I have had an internationally known detective agency digging up information on the medical association." Brinkley would prove to the electorate, he said, that the AMA was running "a plain 'racket,' one of gigantic proportions."

In the fights for his licenses, both lost, powerful friends had availed him nothing. From now on he would make the rules himself. As governor, for starters, he could pack the medical board with his own men. But it was only five weeks until the election, too late even to get his name on the ballot. Political veterans viewed his entering the race as quixotic if not preposterous.

In those few short weeks, however, Brinkley's candidacy would turn the state upside down. It would ignite the biggest uprising by Kansas voters in forty years, and produce strategic innovations that would forever transform the American political campaign.

. . .

Outsiders only dimly familiar with Kansas, then as now, were apt to confuse flat with bland. In fact, ever since its bloody birth in the 1850s, Kansas had specialized in Grand Guignol, in fanatics, demagogues, and plagues. Here abolitionists and slavers had slaughtered each other in the run-up to the Civil War, John Brown had plotted his raid on Harpers Ferry, Carry Nation had turned saloons into kindling with her lively ax, and Populists like Sockless Jerry Simpson and Mary Elizabeth Lease ("raise less corn and more hell!") had lashed farmers into a foam against the "mortgage fiends" back East—all this while biblical doses of grasshoppers, Hessian flies, cinch bugs, blizzards, and tornadoes came sweeping out of the wide sky. Prohibition became law in America in 1918; Kansas passed it in 1881. As psychiatrist Karl A. Menninger, who started his career at the Harvard Medical School, later said of his fellow Kansans: "In abolition, prohibition, Populism, anti-tobacco legislation, Brinkley worship . . . they have gone off the deep end with desperate seriousness."

"It's coming, Ma! Look!"

Darting about the state in his snazzy blue-and-gold plane— previous owner Charles Lindbergh—Brinkley drew the biggest crowds any Kansas politician had ever seen. This wasn't just another droner holding his own lapels; Brinkley put the party in politics with a supersized medicine show, only this time the former Quaker doctor had a big bottle of cure-all for the body politic.

How could a man so recently and comprehensively humiliated win such support? For one thing, there was widespread agreement that the doctor, in his own phrase, had been "kangarooed to kingdom come" by the state medical board. W. G. Clugston, who had covered Kansas politics for years, wrote that even people who didn't like Brinkley believed that the medical board "beyond a doubt, did act as judge, jury and prosecutor, in fact if not in name." He had been lynched, in short, and that discredited the evidence. The same suspicions attached to the *Star*'s vendetta against him. It was so white-hot and went on so long it began to defeat its own purpose.

But voters felt more for the goat-gland man than just sympathy. When he stood on that platform and tore into the government, the AMA, all the powers of darkness out to destroy him, a lot of folks scared to death by the onslaught of the Depression identified with him keenly. They, too, felt threatened with extinction at the hands of the establishment—the bank, the sheriff, "the authorities." Even the drought that struck that summer felt like part of the conspiracy: corn production down by almost half, the papers were saying, "two-thirds of a grape crop, one-half a pear crop, and one-third of the average apple yield—and the livestock industry crippled." The common people were desperate for a savior. Who better than their old friend the doctor with his new crown of thorns?

Cowboy singer Roy Faulkner, KFKB's biggest music star, usually opened the show, ambling onstage with his big hat and his guitar. He sang "Strawberry Roan" and other songs about campfires and prairie dogs. Then Uncle Bob Larkin the fiddle champion took over, the Gospel Quartet four-parted a hymn to the next governor, the Steve Love Orchestra threw in a set, and Minnie and Johnny Boy slipped onstage somewhere between the yodeler and the fortune-teller. Then, while nurses in hospital caps passed through the crowd handing out balloons, noisemakers, and lollipops, a Methodist preacher gave the doctor the biggest buildup since John the Baptist until at last the man of the hour, the "people's candidate," materialized onstage in a white suit with a big sunflower in his buttonhole. It took the crowd forever to quiet down, but when they finally did and he opened his mouth to speak, there came Johnny Boy in his Little Lord Fauntleroy suit bolting from upstage to wrap his arms around his father's leg, and the cheering started all over again. . . .

Morris Fishbein, publicly at least, declined to care. He dismissed Brinkley's run for office as just one more move by "a paranoid type who wanted the limelight and would use every possible technic [*sic*] for getting it." The professional pols still mocked him. But as the days passed they began to realize that Brinkley, so good at circuses, was equally good at promising bread. It wasn't so much the promises themselves—free schoolbooks, lower taxes, old-age pensions, and more rainfall—as the brilliant new ways he was making them. That fancy private plane was more than just great theater; it exponentially increased the number of hands the candidate could pump. And when he wasn't in the air, he was on it. Brinkley fused politics and broad-casting on a scale no one had conceived of before. With all the demands on his time he still spent an average of five hours a day on the radio drenching the electorate with the sound of his voice. (On the rare days he didn't travel, one paper claimed, he was at the micro-phone "from 6:45 in the morning until the hours of darkness come at night.") To reach immigrant voters, he put surrogates on the air speaking in Swedish and German. And the harder he worked, the more fun he seemed to be having. When a prominent newspaperman attacked his candidacy, Brinkley mailed him a goat.

His boisterous innovations as a campaigner earned him levels of attention which for all his fame he had never enjoyed before, both from politicians across the country, who began to study what he was doing, and from the mainstream press. Throughout the 1920s a sort of cultural arrogance had kept papers like the *New York Times* from tracking his adventures much (while giving distinguished professors Voronoff and Steinach reams of respect). That changed now. Not all the coverage was favorable, but the heightened scrutiny had little impact on the voting pool. In state, Brinkley's KFKB still ruled.

Now the backroom boys were getting scared. Leaders of both major parties began to wish they had put a little more thought into choosing their own candidates for governor; right now the biggest question surrounding Democrat Harry Woodring and Republican Frank Haucke was, Which was Tweedledum? Both were novices, both wan bachelors. One liked to knit. All this in disheartening contrast to Brinkley, whose martyrdom at the hands of jealous officials had metastasized into a sort of mass pathology. For Sunday, October 26, nine days before the election, the doctor scheduled a midday rally in a cow pasture outside Wichita. By early afternoon the crowd awaiting him had swollen to thirty or forty thousand. People whooped and pointed every time they saw a buzzard in the blue—"*Here he comes!*"—and finally they were right. The plane circled low several times, driving the crowd to canine levels of excitement, before coasting down onto the grass. As it rolled to a stop it was swarmed. "Don't rush, folks!" a voice hollered through the loudspeakers. "You'll be cut to pieces by the propellers!" Moments later the side hatch swung open and Brinkley, attired in a dark blue suit, purple tie, and white straw hat, stepped out and merged with a "jumping, whooping, yelling, enthusiastic log jam" of fans. Minnie and Johnny Boy struggled along behind. Somebody close heard the little boy crying, "I don't want to shake hands anymore!"

The newly built speaker's platform was solid and commanding, crowned by a small American flag snapping in the prairie wind. As Brinkley waded toward it, "men with crutches, women with goiters, children with eruptions and twisted limbs, all of his constituency, cried out as he went by." Singing started somewhere, and forty thousand throats joined in:

"Oh beautiful for spacious skies/For amber waves of grain . . ."

In the roar that followed, the unseen announcer fought once more to be heard. He introduced Brinkley as a "Moses, who has come to lead us out of the wilderness." But that was the wrong hero, as any child could tell, when the candidate faced the multitude and flung wide his arms.

There would be no Lonesome Cowboy today, no Fenoglio and his Magic Accordion. Not even any talk of politics. This was a Sunday, and on Sundays the doctor confined himself to reflections on the Scripture. For in the end what did the trappings of office matter? "I had rather save a soul," he shouted, "than be president of the United States or even king of the world!"

Then he stood under the beating sun and delivered a sermon on the Passion of Jesus Christ. It included a travelogue of Brinkley's own trip to the Holy Land, his tours of Jerusalem and Palestine, his first sight of Bethlehem—but here his voice broke, for the birthplace of the Lord had moved him profoundly, reminding him as it did of his own humble origins. He had seen the spot where Jesus was jeered by the Philistines. He had visited the temple where Christ had overturned the tables of the moneylenders, men who had traded their shriveled souls for gain.

The doctor paused and slowly drank a glass of water. He placed it back on the stool.

Then suddenly he wheeled about, opened his arms again and cried, "I too have walked up the path Jesus walked to Calvary! I stood in Jesus' tomb! *I know how Jesus felt!*"

A great moan rose from the crowd.

"The men in power wanted to do away with Jesus before the common people woke up! *Are you awake here?*"

They were wide awake.

A space had been reserved for the ill and disfigured by the bottom of the steps, and when at the end he descended from the stage, they were the ones who fell upon him first, crying out for a look, a touch.

When two nights later "Milford's miracle man" held a giant rally at the Wichita Forum, with an audience made up of every age and class ("mink and sealskin . . . rubbed elbows with coats of lesser swank"), the major-party leaders surrendered to panic. At the eleventh hour they huddled with state attorney general William A. Smith, the prosecutor at Brinkley's medical-board hearing (or as the doctor liked to call it, his "Garden of Gethsemane"), to try to think of some way to knock him out of the running. And they found one—they hoped. On November 1, three days before the election, Smith spoke to the press.

The rules regarding write-in votes had been changed, he said. No longer would the "intent of the voter," the standard benightedly set by the Kansas Supreme Court, be sufficient. Instead, the election board now decreed that the doctor's name could be written just one way—J. R. BRINKLEY—for the vote to count.

This flew in the face of American democratic tradition, including the tradition of stealing elections quietly, but with the vote just three days off there was no time to protest. Brinkley spread the word on the radio, rushed out thousands of pencils embossed with the approved spelling of his name, and at his final rallies brought along cheerleaders to drill the crowd:

"J period! R period! . . ."

"It has been said," he cried defiantly, "that the people who vote for Brinkley think the moon is made of green cheese. You have been called numskulls [sic]. But I want to tell my opponents that the greatest handwriting contest that has ever been pulled off in the nation will come to pass on Election Day. Right now there are Germans, Russians, Lithuanians and others who have little knowledge of the English language, staying up nights to learn how to write the name of J. R. Brinkley!"

When the big day dawned, nothing was clear but the weather. The resident fortune-teller and "people's psychologist" on KFKB announced that Dr. Brinkley would win by a landslide, but most others wouldn't even speculate. As a typical editorial put it, "[O]bservers who have guessed community results with uncanny accuracy for more than a third of a century are stumped."

"J period! R period! . . ."

All day the chant continued, issuing from every loudspeaker and megaphone Brinkley Boosters could lay their hands on. Turnout was heavy. "When the voting returns began coming in on election night," W. G. Clugston reported, "there was plenty of alarm, for the early returns showed Brinkley running far ahead. . . . So many citizens had written his name on their ballots the counting officials couldn't put him out of the running, not even when they put their heads together and made that the chief objective of the count."

The tally took twelve days. The final results:

Woodring (D): 217,171
Haucke (R): 216,920
Brinkley (Independent): 183,278

But this total did not include the ballots with *Doctor Brinkley*, *Doc Brinkly* and other variants, all of which were disqualified—to say nothing of the freethinkers who liked him for lieutenant governor, U.S. senator, Kansas supreme court justice, and other posts. The doctor was so popular he even carried three counties in Oklahoma.

How large was the disqualified vote? The *Des Moines Register*, a leading out-of-state newspaper, viewed it this way:

> Were it not for the fact that one out of six of his supporters failed to write his name correctly on the ballot, Dr. J. R. Brinkley, the goat-gland specialist whose license was revoked in September by the state medical board, would today be governor-elect of Kansas. Brinkley garnered more than 183,000 votes, without having his name on the ballot, and it is estimated that from 30,000 to 50,000 others intended to vote for him but spoiled their ballots by mistake.
>
> This phenomenon is without precedent. In 1924, when the famous William Allen White ran as an independent candidate for governor of Kansas, he received only 149,000 votes, even though his name was on the ballot. Brinkley, who entered the campaign late and who campaigned by radio and traveled by airplane, drew larger crowds in Kansas than any previous political speaker, not excepting Roosevelt, Bryan, Wilson or Al Smith.

If ever an election cried out for a recount, this was it, and not just because of support for the goat-gland man. Republican candidate Haucke had finished in a dead heat with Woodring, a mere 251 votes behind. But instead of starting a fracas in court, as everyone expected, Haucke and his party vanished like the dew. The risk was too great, they decided, that a recount would crown Brinkley governor.

That left it up to the doctor himself. His backers begged him to fight. That last-minute rule about write-in votes had been a naked abuse of Smith's authority, they said. It would surely collapse on appeal.

Yet in the end the doctor decided not to challenge the results. As W. G. Clugston explained: "Brinkley's political advisers persuaded him not to institute a contest and demand a recount. They told him it would be better sportsmanship to accept the decision . . . and then to run again in the next election when he would have ample time to get his name printed on the ballots. To make their arguments convincing, they pointed out that when Arthur Capper first ran for governor 18 years before he was defeated by only 52 votes, and didn't start a contest—and that two years later when Capper ran again he was elected by a landslide, and had stayed in the governor's office and the United States Senate continuously from that time on."

So the doctor agreed to take the high road and wait two years. But Kansans across the spectrum knew he'd been robbed. Even Harry Woodring, the man sworn in as governor, later admitted that "there were sufficient votes" to elect Brinkley "had all invalidated ballots been counted." Eventually Haucke acknowledged it, too.

As it was, the doctor's campaign accomplished much. It proved, for one thing, that if a man behaves outrageously enough, disgrace is impossible. But it was in his fusion of politics and radio—his virtuosic manipulation of the airwaves to win votes—and his dazzling use of the airplane that its lasting impact lay. He had just run the first campaign of the modern age. Huey Long took notes, Pappy O'Daniel in Texas, everybody.

Even so, in the fall of 1930 the doctor looked less like a pioneer than a loser. In the space of a few months he had lost the election, lost KFKB, and lost his medical license. Now he had nothing.

Except another brainwave.

32

Long before they rescinded his license, Brinkley had despised the fusspots at the Federal Radio Commission. He hated their fuddy-duddy regulations, especially the one that limited most stations to a mere five thousand watts. A rule like that, he believed, could have but one purpose: to strangle genius.

Now the answer came to him, perfect and complete.

Mexico.

Why not build a radio station south of the border, just across the Rio Grande, where the American government couldn't get at him? If he could sell the Mexican authorities on the idea, he could put whatever he liked on the air and blow it over half the Western world.

What made him think of this nobody knows. Perhaps his inglorious ministint in the military, when he was stationed near the border town of El Paso, returned to mind. (Texas did have the best cold beer he'd ever tasted.) Or maybe he remembered how much his old friend Harry Chandler liked Mexico, so much that he had invaded it with a private army trying to annex the Baja peninsula. Or maybe Brinkley had got wind of a small American-owned station already operating over the border: XED, aka "The Voice of Two Republics," which had been on the air just a few weeks. Broadcasting from the northeastern town of Reynosa, it played Tex-Mex music at a decorous ten thousand watts and wasn't causing anyone any trouble—a setup Brinkley could have only viewed as an opportunity squandered.

Up to now, America had troubled itself over Mexican radio only once. It happened during the First World War, when German U-boats were having a suspiciously easy time torpedoing American shipping in the Pacific. Intelligence reports suggested that a spy with a wireless was signaling enemy submarines from somewhere in the Mexican hills, and U.S. Treasury agent Al Scharff—former miner, rustler, counterfeiter, and soldier in the Mexican army—was dispatched to track him down. Along with a Pina Indian guide named Red Slippers and a small team of mercenaries, Scharff entered the desert. A few days later they pinpointed the radio in a cave in the mountains of Cabo Lobos. As dawn broke, he and his men crawled toward it through the creosote bushes and prickly pear, and in the gun battle that followed the Germans were killed and the transmitter destroyed. Then Scharff stuffed the cave with dynamite and blew it up.

That episode aside, the U.S. government thought of Mexican radio as a joke, an oxymoron. When Mexico City tried to negotiate the sharing of commercial bandwidths in the mid-1920s, Washington scoffed, tossed a few to Canada, and took the rest. No wonder, then, that in February 1931, when Dr. Brinkley visited their capital city to pitch his scheme, Mexican authorities embraced him like a lost relative. They were delighted to cooperate on a project that promised (1) to bring a lot of cash to the northern provinces and (2) to wreak havoc on "the imperialistic aerial designs of the United States." Brinkley and his new host country would be partners in revenge.

In March the doctor sold KFKB to a Wichita insurance company and made plans to move south. He wasn't quitting Kansas altogether. "Brinkley has served notice that he will run [for governor in 1932]," the *New York Times* reported. "He will maintain his residence [in] Milford and operate his Mexican broadcasting station by remote control. Political leaders see no way of heading him off." Even his clinic in Milford, though he couldn't practice there himself, remained open under the aegis of two staff quacks, Drs. Owensby and Dragoo.

The doctor still had not decided where to locate along the two-thousand-mile Mexican border. Then one day he got a letter from A. B. Easterling, secretary of the Del Rio, Texas, chamber of commerce. Situated 150 miles west of San Antonio, Del Rio touted itself as "the

Queen City of the Rio Grande" and "the Wool and Mohair Capital of the Nation," when in truth it was just another dusty little town made desperate by the Great Depression. "We certainly hope that you will at least pay us a visit," Easterling wrote. "The Mayor of Villa Acuna [the town facing Del Rio over the river] has already assured the Mexican consul that their city will furnish, free, adequate land for the purpose of erecting your station."

Brinkley flew down to take a look. He liked what he saw. The celebrated Judge Roy Bean—like the doctor, a lover of liquor and lucre, and a law unto himself—had died in Del Rio in 1903. The town had a proven tolerance for tall tales: half the population believed in Pecos Bill the way kids did Santa Claus. As for competition, according to a local historian, "the only radio Del Rio had seen was a homemade set of copper coils wound around an oatmeal carton." He would own the place.

Brinkley crossed the international bridge into Villa Acuna, a lively little town with casinos, two movie houses, and a good bullring, and signed the papers there. Issued on April 30, his Mexican radio license came with fifty thousand watts to play with, ten times what he'd had before. An official who helped draft the contract described it as "a blanket concession" giving Brinkley "absolute freedom in control of the station."

Construction of the new $350,000 "border blaster"—call letters XER—began that summer on a ten-acre site outside town. The work went fast. Told on a tour that he would need custom-designed transmitter tubes, Brinkley took a roll from his pocket and peeled off thirty-six thousand-dollar bills.

All the while Morris Fishbein was watching, metaphorically at least, through binoculars.

When letters and phone calls failed, he flew to Texas determined to kill the project. Others were, too. Officials at the U.S. embassy in Mexico, under orders from the State Department, were searching for some way, any way, to stop it. Dope smugglers they were used to, gunrunners, cattle rustlers, illegal aliens floundering through the water trying to get from the poverty and gila monsters south of the border to the poverty and gila monsters on the other side. But this was not in the manual.

In Austin, Fishbein brought his gale-force eloquence before the state medical board hoping to get Brinkley's license pulled. To no avail: Fishbein's quack was their golden goose. The editor returned to Chicago undecided about what to do next—to be greeted by the extraordinary news that others had succeeded where he had not. Under heavy pressure from the State Department, the Mexican government had halted construction of XER.

For a few weeks Fishbein savored the victory. Then it began to slip away. The moment he heard of the shutdown, Brinkley cabled the most powerful politician he knew, his old friend Vice President Charles Curtis, for help: "I am moving to have an investigation made in Mexico City and uncover the prime movers in this plot coming from Washington and expose the whole sordid mess. . . .

"The people of Kansas feel that you are interested in fair play and that you will have an investigation made of this so the newspapers of Kansas can tell the people just what is being done against Dr. J. R. Brinkley of Milford, Kansas, his wife and baby. STOP."

Curtis was a political fixer of wide experience. As majority leader of the Senate, he had been known for his skill in brokering deals. Somebody called him one of the great "whisperers" on Capitol Hill: "Whenever he took his favorite pose, with a short fat arm coiled around another Senator's shoulders, the Press Gallery got busy." Nowadays, however, Curtis was unhappily mired in the second spot, shunned by Hoover and "gazing through a film of what might have been tears at his old seat on the [Senate] floor." Inspired in part by his plight, the Gershwins were about to premiere *Of Thee I Sing,* a Broadway musical in which woefully underoccupied Vice President Alexander Throttlebottom can't even get a library card.

Thanks to Hoover's paralytic response to the Depression, Curtis was not only idle; he was political dead meat. But now as he read Brinkley's telegram he had a rush of hope. By rescuing the widely popular doctor, maybe he could redeem himself in the eyes of Kansas voters, maybe win back some of those infuriated farmers who used to be his friends. Maybe he could save his career.

Curtis still had connections, and he knew where the bodies were buried. Now he eagerly went to work defeating the efforts of his own State Department. He followed up a bland letter ("Mr. Curtis . . . hope[s] the Department may find it possible not to place additional obstructions in Dr. Brinkley's way") with some arm-twisting both in Washington and at the U.S. embassy in Mexico. Just how ugly things got isn't clear, but a nascent prosecution of Brinkley for mail fraud was apparently nipped in the process. Fishbein had long been agitating to have the charges brought. Missouri's health commissioner, too, was urging that Brinkley's promoting his "gland racket" by form letter was a crime: "He might as well say that he can cut out my eye and then cut out your eye and put it into my head and that it will grow fast and that I can see through it. . . . Brinkley is a fraud of the most dangerous type and the United States authorities in Kansas will be derelict in their duty to the public if they do not cause his arrest for using the mails to defraud." Prosecution had appeared imminent: two postal inspectors took notes throughout Brinkley's appearance before the FRC. But once Curtis intervened there wasn't another peep about it. Instead, the "great whisperer" got Brinkley's Mexico scheme back on track.

Within weeks two three-hundred-foot towers were completed, not far from a fountain with a stone egret spitting water at the sky. Over the door of the studio, the station's call letters, XER, were chiseled in lightning bolts. Inside, engineering whiz James Weldon created a den of wonders. "The transmitter room was the classic science-fiction-movie idea of a radio," a visitor said, "with rack after rack of black, ominous panels, covered with meters, water valves, buttons, lights and glass portholes for looking in on the expensive circuits."

In October 1931, the Sunshine Station Between the Nations made its debut. Del Rio celebrated with XER Gala Week, a jubilee crowned by a feast in honor of the goat-gland surgeon and his wife. The evening's entertainment featured Tex-Mex singers, a commemorative poem supplied by the chamber of commerce, and Mrs. Brinkley's sister in a solo ballet.

Any reveler who happened to wander outside had a clear view of the station's gigantic towers rising side by side into the night sky. Along the wires eerie green lights crackled and spat.

33

One night early on in the Depression, a kitchen worker came around a corner and found fifty men fighting over a barrel of restaurant garbage. With misery at that pitch, the national suicide rate was rising sharply. Many people were getting sick, especially in families without a full-time worker—and for a time that was most American households.

Poverty and fear worked on the mind like weevils. Some men lucky enough to find a job were frightened to take it, afraid they wouldn't do it properly, afraid of being fired again. The women's fashion industry jettisoned the streetwise flapper for a fluffier, softer look, a move some saw as an effort to shore up battered masculine pride. But how their women dressed (the few who could afford new clothes) made little difference to the millions of men riven by failure—failure they carried all too often into the bedroom.

And that meant boom times for John Brinkley, M.D. It was yet another miracle of his career that when the 1920s zeitgeist collapsed, taking most of its fads and fortunes with it, he remained brilliantly afloat. Had it not been for the Depression, in fact, the rejuvenation craze might have burned out sooner. As it was, what brought him success in the age of prosperity would lift him even higher in the age of despair. Quacks are always lavish with promises of hope, and in the hell of the Depression, a lot of people went where the hope was.

All the rejuvenationists, the sincere ones included, got a new lease on life. Serge Voronoff had lately gone partners with nonsinging diva

Ganna Walska (married at last to Harold McCormick) in a beauty shop on the Champs-Elysées. But lotions and creams hadn't stolen his focus. Indeed, he was higher on chimps than ever. Thanks to gland transplantation, he was saying now, science was close to creating "a race of supermen" and superwomen, too. The female had "a more complicated physique," so the problem had taken longer to solve, but he was now confident that by grafting three monkey glands, the thyroid, pituitary, and ovarian, he could achieve results comparable to those for men. Soon women, too, would live to 150.

Steinach's method remained popular as well. New rejuvenationists like Dr. Karl Doppler of Vienna and Dr. Harry Benjamin of New York had their variants and vogues. Each new face reignited the old debate. "The passage of physical time is inexorable and irreversible. No one can think of controlling it," said Dr. Alexis Carrel, a Nobel Prize winner at the Rockefeller Institute. But for every Carrel, there was a Dr. Eusebio A. Hernandez of Paris, who in a speech at the Harvard Medical School declared that not only was greater longevity possible but also the prevention of death was within reach—witness the "experiments of Professor J. P. Heymans, who preserved life in an isolated head for three hours." While clergymen deplored this obsession with extending life, reminding congregations it was the afterlife that mattered, Dr. Anna Ingerman was telling the League of Advertising Women that glands "might almost be called the seat of the soul."

Stymied in his pursuit of Brinkley, at least for now, Fishbein turned his attention elsewhere. Quackery was such a hot stock these days—four AMA chemists were working full-time just analyzing bogus tonics—that he produced a new book, *Fads and Quackery in Healing,* with exposés of the latest rackets, including aerotherapy, autohemic therapy, and astral therapy; biodynamochromatic diagnosis and therapy (patient faces east or west and practices "rithmo-chrome breathing" while his abdomen is thumped under colored lights); Christos (tonics designed to rid the body of impurities and sin at the same time);

geotherapy (pressing the patient's body with "little pads of earth"), limpio comerology (health achieved by eating "Q-33 and Q-34"), pathiatry, poropathy, sanatology, spectrocromism (bathing patient in colored lights, palette tailored to the disease); tropo-therapy, Vita-O-Path (thirty-six quackeries rolled into one), and zonotherapy, which "heals disease in one zone by pressing on others"—a toothache on the right side, for example, was treated with a small wire wrapped around the second toe of the left foot.

As a tour of the human imagination, it was better than Jules Verne, but it didn't begin to suggest the full scope of the problem— including the fact that Fishbein had few weapons to fight it with. "The A.M.A. actually has no legal powers," he elsewhere explained, "no punitive powers, and no authority to stop anyone from practicing medicine of any kind, no matter how questionable its validity. It controls quackery and exploitation of the public only by a program of public education." As the war on Brinkley had already shown, state and federal law was impossibly porous regarding the criminal liability of quacks. Short of shooting a patient on Main Street, a physician was almost untouchable. He could be sued in civil court, of course, but this put the onus on the victim, who risked throwing good money (if he had it) after bad in a vain attempt to win damages. As for those gizmos and gadgets, with their twirling lights and wires to nowhere, they were all legal. For decades, a friend later said, "Morris kept up the battle as the lone voice in the wilderness" to get a law banning fraudulent medical devices on the books.

Fishbein even faced resistance from the very people he was trying to help. Colleagues might applaud his zeal. (Thorek wrote to him in the spring of 1930: "Your relentless fight against these 'pests' should immortalize you.") But that didn't mean that average folks liked to see him coming. The quacks brought the good news: It works! He brought the bad news. Which did a sick person want to hear?

Given all this, Fishbein through sheer force of personality scored more wins than anyone had a right to expect.

Henry Junius Schireson was perhaps the most notorious plastic-surgery quack of the day, spreading pain and disfigurement as he shifted from state to state. Despite his track record, and a bribery conviction in Pittsburgh, he used the audacity of an A-list shark to build a prestigious clientele that included Broadway star Fanny Brice. Then one day a young woman came to him for treatment of a shoulder burn. He offered to straighten her bowlegs while she was there. As a result, both had to be amputated at the knee.

Fishbein made her case a cause célèbre. In 1930, thanks to his steady pot banging, Schireson was found guilty of gross malpractice and driven out of Illinois. When he tried to relocate in Ohio, Fishbein was there to greet him. Wherever he tried to set up shop, the editor poisoned the well, till at last Schireson floundered east to Philadelphia, bankruptcy, and prison.

Others Fishbein harmed or ruined included Percival Lemon Clark, a self-styled "sanatologist" who was a pet of Henry Ford; the flamboyant dentist Painless Parker, who had legally changed his name to Painless so he could use the word in his advertising; and John Paul Fernel, designer of a "sleeping brassiere" that supposedly shrank oversized busts. Fishbein never let up. The punishing pace (a friend called his metabolism "a cosmic accident") led to what were vaguely described as "nervous breakdowns" along the way. As a colleague recalled it, "[O]n at least four occasions he had an acute syncope while making public addresses"—that is, a loss of consciousness, probably from a shortage of oxygen to the brain. Fishbein dismissed it as exhaustion and pressed on. He rarely went to a doctor himself, trusting instead to his own random stash of pills.

Still writing for the *Mercury*, he suggested a story to Mencken in 1931 about the mania for antiseptics spawned by Listerine: "An old eclectic physician made the terse statement that if the rectum had teeth, we would undoubtedly have special brushes and chemicals for keeping them in a sterile condition." Mostly, though, he kept bashing alternative medicine. When he learned that a Christian Science healer had withheld insulin from a diabetic six-year-old who then died, Fish-bein found a judge with diabetes and had the Christian Scientist arrested for murder. But the law in those days didn't cover the case—the first death-by-bad-doctoring conviction wouldn't come till the 1960s—so the charges didn't stick.

34

Out of the limestone catacombs a king snake slithers, moving like a whip in slow motion. Gorgeously banded in black and salmon, it slides through underground gullies and crevices upward toward the light. The ancient murals it passes are black and salmon too, and orange-red and caramel and white. One depicts a towering white shaman, his torso fantastically stretched, showering small black figures who are upside down, representing the dead. . . .

W e played near the station," guitarist Juan Raul Rodriguez said. "We slept near the station, we never left it. . . . At night you heard the beautiful music everywhere and you saw flashing lights dancing along the wires, just like the angels in heaven."

Brinkley stayed mostly on the Texas side of the river, broadcasting from a snug little studio over Del Rio's J. C. Penney store. Thumbing his nose at U.S. authorities, he made regular visits to Milford and programmed from there as well, using a phone line that bounced his voice through his Mexican transmitter. Broadcasting via international telephone wasn't against the law because no one had thought to do it before.

XER was a dream come true. During the week of January 11–16, 1932, the station reaped 27,717 listener letters from across North

America. Del Rio became famous overnight, its businesses were saved, and the doctor "ravished the town" by spending generously on civic improvements, including a new library. Not everyone loved him. Across the river a principled minority was incensed that XER, though built on Mexican soil, was owned and operated by Americans broadcasting almost entirely in English. "The protesting patriots," as *La Prensa* called them, resented "the tolerance shown this propaganda of Yankee imperialism . . . and they have sent a copy of their complaint to the Ministry of the Interior."

But as Brinkley liked to say, "I get fat off my enemies," even when he wasn't trying to. When as a sop to the protesters he added a third "directional" tower to block his broadcasts in most of Mexico, it had the happy effect of multiplying his effective wattage north. With the consent of Mexico City, he upped the juice to 150,000 watts in January 1932. Then in August, to the rising dismay of the U.S. government, he got another bump to half a million watts, and then a million—a million watts!—making XER far and away the most powerful radio station on the planet. A technician there now reported that the transmitter "makes the hair on your arms stand up." Locals said the signal was so strong it turned on car headlights, made their bedsprings hum, and sent Brinkley's voice wandering in and out of other people's telephone conversations.

That voice, dropping as the gentle rain, was now heard in every state in the Union and at least fifteen foreign countries. Parked at 735 kilocycles in the center of the broadcast band, it sometimes big-footed even the mightiest American stations, like Atlanta's WSB and Chicago's WGN. A Montreal station two thousand miles away reported chronic interference from XER. On clear nights Brinkley reached Alaska, skipped across to Finland, was picked up by ships on the Java Sea. In later years Russian spies reportedly used the station to help them learn English.

The rude reach of XER made some Americans hopping mad. After a hard day's work, a lot of folks tuning in for Amos and Andy or Charlie McCarthy didn't want to hear about testicles instead. But while they railed at "Mexico's radio outlaw" and the "bootlegger of the air," others reacted differently—for along with all the blarney and nefarious advice came some first-class Tex-Mex and hillbilly music, music millions had never heard before, music they knew nothing about. Music they loved.

Some of the performers dated back to KFKB days, like golden-throated Roy Faulkner. But the talent pool soon widened dramatically as musicians began streaming in from across the South and West. The *Grand Ole Opry* was a great regional show, but it couldn't match the border blaster's phenomenal penetration—and the national networks, CBS and NBC, didn't have much truck with hillbillies.

Brinkley threw wide the door. Patsy Montana (a sparkling yodeler, soon to become the first million-selling female country artist with "I Want to Be a Cowboy's Sweetheart"), Red Foley, Gene Autry, Jimmie Rodgers, the Pickard Family, Cowboy Slim Rinehart: these and many more bellied up to microphones crowned with the XER lightning bolts. Del Rio became known as "Hillbilly Hollywood" for the wealth of country-music talent it attracted, thus turning Brinkley (who personally preferred organ music) into a sort of accidental titan of pop culture. As Bill C. Malone wrote in his definitive *Country Music, U.S.A.*, it was the goat-gland king who "popularized hillbilly music throughout the United States and laid the basis for country music's great popularity in the late 40s and early 50s."

Not all his stars were musicians. The doc had a canny eye for talent of all types, and before long the station's top "mail puller" (after himself) was a hard-eyed bottle-blonde with a passing resemblance to Mae West. Her name was Rose Dawn, aka the Patroness of the Sacred Order of Maya: "Let the Mayans help you find yourself. . . ."

Whatever goat glands didn't fix, Rose could. She peddled a self-help package that included step-by-step directions for "obtaining your desires," also a guaranteed way to increase your income, plus how to develop personal magnetism, all for $4.98. Or she would send you a perfume that accomplished the same thing. Or say you didn't have the $4.98; Rose promised to pray for anyone who sent her a dollar. She also made the on-air prediction that Dr. Brinkley's personality and good works would put him in the White House, a proposition accepted by many as proof of her divine gifts.

Off duty Rose liked to cruise the streets of Del Rio in her pink Chrysler with green trim, accompanied by her tall dark smoothie of a boyfriend, the astrologer-mentalist Koran. Gossips in Del Rio guessed she was Brinkley's mistress, too, but there was never any evidence of it. He wasn't the type.

Up to now Brinkley had broadcast only advertisements for himself, but the success of Rose Dawn caused him to reconsider. With hucksters too nasty, salacious, or just plain crazy for American radio begging him for airtime, he decided to give them a chance—at $1,700 an hour. Suddenly XER gained a chorus of voices jabbering the praises of Crazy Water Crystals, electric bow ties, rupture cures, "genuine simulated" diamonds, tomato plants, life insurance, live poultry, and an array of religious items including Last Supper tablecloths and autographed pictures of Christ. Somebody peddled a windup John the Baptist doll: turn the key, and he walked around till his head fell off.

Toe-tapping tunes mixed with raucous hard sell: AM radio was crawling out of the ooze.

35

Now, of course, every screwball on the continent wanted a border blaster of his own, and for a time in the early thirties Mexico was dealing them out like cards. In 1932 Norman Baker, after his Iowa station was shut down by the Federal Radio Commission, built XENT in Nuevo Laredo, licensed at 150,000 watts. He painted the exterior walls of his studio bright purple and started an on-air feud with Brinkley. Country singer Hank Thompson recalled it as "a slugfest like Jack Benny and Fred Allen."

Other stations sprang up—XERB in Rosarito Beach, XELO in Cuidad Juarez, XEG in Monterrey, XEPN in Piedras Negras—each with a sister town in Texas delighted to have it there. "[T]he pickings are so good that radio stations are sticking up like oil derricks," said the *Chicago Daily News,* though Brinkley's remained by far the biggest and best known. In 1932 when the FRC banned "spooks"— mind readers, astrologers, fortune-tellers, yogis, mystics, "psychists," and seers—they knew just where to go. Overnight the Mexican border was crawling with turbaned individuals once suckled by shamans or teleported from Dimension 9. In the town of Eagle Pass, Texas, just over the river from one station, so many spooks collected that they formed a baseball team. They had time to play, since their psychic powers were frequently farmed out to somebody else. A former San Antonio reporter fallen on hard times found himself ghosting for a spook, answering listener letters at three cents each—advising people to marry, divorce, buy, sell as the mood struck him.

Other refugees from the United States were victims of religious persecution. The Federal Radio Commission in those days forbade evangelists from soliciting donations on the air, an antediluvian scruple that put some big personalities on the highway south. The granddaddies of today's televangelists honed their craft on outlaw radio. Cowboy evangelist Dallas Turner, Reverend Eugene Smith ("an expert on the Second Coming"), Frederick Eikerenkoetter II (Reverend Ike)—all rejuvenated their careers pitching and praying in Dr. Brinkley's radio tent.

Eventually eleven border blasters stood along the banks of the Rio Grande, radiating in toto at least seven hundred thousand more watts than all the U.S. stations put together. Dirty country songs, routines Mae West couldn't get away with in the States, that was just for starters. "Preachers fought off Satan right on mike," one veteran recalled, "screamed about killing the rich and eating them." Ladies' man Norman Baker reportedly installed a bed next to his studio mike so he could pitch his cancer cure while having sex. At Piedras Negras, a quarrel between the station's U.S. and Mexican owners came to an end when somebody—it was never clear who—blew up the transmitter. All this while back-country boogie, western swing, lonesome cowboys, comedy acts, San Antonio's Mexican Symphony Orchestra, Woody Guthrie, and human doorways to heretofore unknown faiths were flooding America like bucket-wash:

> *I went to see my Cindy Lou*
> *For pleasure I was seekin'*
> *I missed her mouth and kissed her nose*
> *And the gol-dern thing was leakin'*
> *Get along home, Cindy Cindy*
> *Get along home, Cindy Cindy . . .*

As for the sponsors who made it all possible, they transformed customers' lives with products like Kolorbak hair dye (which caused lead poisoning), Lash Lure (blindness), Radithor ("Certified Radioactive Water"), and Koremlu, later described by investigators as "a depilatory made from rat poison." Lysol was touted as "a safe douche."

Late in the summer of 1932 a bunch of Mexican quacks, emboldened and inspired by the new border blasters, held a convention of their own in the north-central town of Villa Juarez. The most prominent among them were Nino Fidencio (the nation's premier "banned saint") and Nina Lupe, who trafficked in chameleons' brains. As a side attraction, an army commander revealed how to pay fines "by magical arts without losing a penny."

No doubt that last was extremely popular, times being what they were.

"Dr. and Mrs. Brinkley have helped you and are now asking you to help them because their expenses are great and they have a hard struggle making ends meet and you do your friends a great favor when you send them to Dr. and Mrs. B. . . ."

It seemed that everyone had it tough. But while the doctor suffered, or pretended to, his radio talks were gaining a new breadth and confidence. From time to time he departed from his usual wallet-emptying medico-religious palaver and pastoral bloviations to deliver quasi-Emersonian lectures with titles like "Highway Safety," "The Mormons," "Tribute to Mother," and "Idiosyncrasy." He preached a sermon every Sunday: "Find God and be happy. It is the only way. . . ."

To his wife: "I'm on top of the world!"

36

In August 1932 an editorial in the *Baltimore Sun* recalled how Brinkley's run for the Kansas governorship two years back had "jarred the kidneys of every literate person in the state." The piece was unsigned, but the tone of morbid relish is characteristic of Mencken, and its peroration, too: "In 1930 Brinkley came near winning without even having his name on the ballot. This year his name will be on the ballot. Let us offer up a prayer for Kansas."

With crop prices down 90 percent, some Kansas farmers the previous winter had burned their wheat to keep warm. Now as the governor's race of '32 loomed, a straw poll by the *Wichita Beacon* found Brinkley four times more popular than the incumbent. After William Allen White, editor of the *Emporia Gazette,* called Brinkley Boosters the "moronic underworld" of the state, they happily crowned themselves "Old Bill White's Morons, Illiterates and Underworld Characters," and meetings got even louder and prouder.

Once burned, however, the doctor was nervous about his chances. This, combined with the wonderful fact that, according to his engineer James Weldon, Brinkley was "an easy mark for the sales pitches of others," led to his trolling for reassurance in some out-of-the-way places.

"The vibrational forces which you are trying to obtain on [election day] will be perfect for you," wrote numerologist Floyd R. Underwood of Bloomington, Illinois, in response to the doctor's query, a prediction based in part on Brinkley's "ego number" of four. A stargazer in Crystal Bay, Minnesota, was equally sanguine. When

Brinkley consulted astrologer Evangeline Adams of New York City, America's most fashionable seer, she gave him a mild scolding at first: "I still feel that you expect too much from Astrology, and that you do not realize that it is only one factor in determining what will happen. . . . For instance, if you choose to throw yourself in front of an express train on one of your lucky days, it will kill you just the same as though it were one of your bad ones." Her next letter, though, was more encouraging. "I find that the powerful planet Jupiter will be more friendly to you than it has been for about twelve years. . . . The fact that this planet is on your Midheaven . . . certainly does promise something very much out of the ordinary which will affect you in a most satisfactory manner, and which may have a bearing on both state and national affairs. . . .

"I am inclined to the belief of our greatest showman, P. T. Barnum, who was of the opinion that every knock is a boost, and that any book your first wife may write will not do any material harm, although let us hope that it will not be published at a time when either Saturn or Uranus are unfriendly to your Mercury."

This last reference was to recent rowdy remarks by the former Sally Wike, now remarried and living in Illinois. Still seething at the doctor's refusal through the years to recognize her extralegal right to some of his money, she had launched a guerrilla war on his gubernatorial campaign. Lately she had paid calls on Governor Woodring and Alf Landon (the presumptive Republican nominee) to give them ammunition and was threatening to write a book about Brinkley's early years. Evangeline Adams asked for Sally's date of birth in order to determine "whether she will really be able to hurt you in the end."

Brinkley's campaign for the governorship was going full bore by June, bringing with it more tireless experiments in self-promotion. This year, mixed in with the airplane hops, he sometimes arrived at rallies in the backseat of a regal, golden brown sixteen-cylinder convertible, driven by a beaming Roy Faulkner with a cavalcade of horn honkers strung out behind. The biggest of these was a gaily painted

Chevrolet truck called "Ammunition Train No. 1." It was equipped with a tailgate stage and loudspeakers, and surmounted by a "five-mile horn"—square mouthed, four feet across, and capable of delivering a blast that could send people running outdoors as if it were the Last Trumpet.

But his speeches played lower notes than in 1930, and in a different key. Often he timed his caravan to roll into town around sunset. The portable stage came down, Roy Faulkner warbled into the twilight, and a jazz combo followed with a mournful "St. Louis Blues" ("I hate to see that evening sun go down . . . / 'Cause my lovin' baby, she done left this town . . ."). By then it was night. As the musicians cleared off, a single cone of light appeared downstage center, into which stepped Reverend Samuel Cookson of Milford to introduce the candidate (something he did so often and so well he was later censured by his Methodist brethren for doing the work of the devil). Brinkley replaced him, melting out of the shadows, dressed in a white linen suit and soft straw hat. He seated himself at the microphone and then (to quote a reporter from Topeka) in the "dim religious light . . . Doc Brinkley purr[ed] into the mike as gently as though he were offering a lady a cup of tea, [or] offering to lend a friend $10 till pay day. . . . As a talker who gets his idea over to his listeners and makes it soak in, Doc Brinkley has some magic that [not] only is different but is tremendously effective."

The doctor knew that his crucifixion road show, so galvanizing two years before, would no longer be fresh or even relevant. *Charm* was the watchword now. (Razzed repeatedly during one speech by a man going "ba-a-a, ba-a-a," the doctor said pleasantly, "Do that a little louder. I may be able to use you.") Yet martyrdom for Brinkley was always more than just a pose, and a close observer could see the stigmata still. If anything his sense of persecution had only increased since the last election, along with persecution's near relation, paranoia.

He spoke publicly and privately of assassination plots against him and—with the Lindbergh case making headlines—of supposed threats to kidnap his son. He claimed Governor Woodring had "extended executive clemency to certain inmates" in prison if they would murder him before election day. To his manager Ernest A. Dewey he wrote: "What I want, Dewey, is a bullet-proof vest that goes down below the waist line and protects both front, back and sides, and fits up around the neck because I am not going to be any too safe along in October and November this year, facing some of these crazy mobs. . . . This is to be kept an absolute secret. In your negotiations you should never let the people you are negotiating with have any idea as to who wants it or anything about it. Should it become known that I am wearing one, the fellow would aim his bullet toward my head or some unprotected spot. . . ." Dewey came back with a size forty vest supplied by a detective agency, assuring Brinkley that it was "exactly like the one worn by Al Capone, and therefore, ought to be the best available."

Throughout the summer and into the fall the doctor darted back and forth between campaign appearances and marathon appeals on the radio. Though he no longer owned it, KFBI in Milford—successor to KFKB—gave him generous airtime, and one day this ping-ponging from stage to studio to stage sparked his next eureka moment.

"I just realized," he wrote one of his advisers, "that I could put a talking machine on my truck and it could stop in a lot of little towns where I would not appear in person to make speeches and, of course, the truck would attract the crowd and the man in charge, after the crowd was collected, could play some of the records and I could make a speech or two from the record. . . .

"I think it the biggest idea I have had. What do you think?"

Thus the sound truck entered American politics, all talking, all singing:

> Surgeon J. R. Brinkley has talents rare and great
> And occupies the limelight in our Sunflower State
> He keeps us all in wonder what he will bring us next
> In surgery or statecraft, or lessons from a text!

Feeling frisky and increasingly confident, the doctor scheduled a campaign stop in the heart of enemy territory. In the summer twilight Ammunition Train No. 1 sat parked on the edge of a baseball field in Emporia, hometown of his noisiest adversary, William Allen White.

It was a nice night. The late August air, often harsh, was breathable for once, and the park lights were off to keep the gnats away. From a nearby outdoor roller rink came the whiz and rumble of skates and cries of glee. Through the crowd awaiting Brinkley—more gawkers than boosters probably, but a gratifying turnout—popcorn, peanut, and ice-cream vendors wormed their way.

Where was he?

Roy Faulkner, the blues orchestra, all the opening acts had come and gone. Now the baby spot was supposed to snap on, that tantalizing pool of light waiting for the great man to fill it. Time passed. The night deepened. Heads went up, looking around for the moon.

Then came what a member of the crowd described as "a weird voice cleaving the darkness."

"I just hope Mr. White and the *Kansas City Star* keep on ripping me wide open because if they do I am going to get at least 500,000 votes next November!" cried the voice.

Was it Brinkley? The audience muttered and peered.

"The American Medical Association ran me off of a 5,000-watt station and I bounced up in Mexico!" the voice continued. "They never will keep Dr. Brinkley off the air, for if Dr. Brinkley cannot broadcast on the continent he will buy a ship and construct a half-million-watt broadcasting station on it and cruise out beyond the twelve-mile limit! And then what I say will be aplenty!"

Brinkley gave the whole speech that way. The prankish arrogance that had brought him to the enemy camp deserted him at the last minute, apparently replaced by fear he might be shot, for he wound up delivering his message of defiance from the shadows in his bullet-proof vest. ("He came and went like a wraith, without handshaking, without personal contact with the common people, a man of mystery!") He made no other stop like it.

Weird as it was, it still agitated William Allen White, but then Brinkley always made him a little crazy. "Are we going to bow our heads after the election," he ranted to his readers, "bow in shame that the intelligent, patriotic people of this State did not have the sense or the courage to avert this disgrace? Shall Kansans be greeted by a gibing b-a-a-a, the cry of the billy goat, when they walk the streets of other States?

"Save Kansas!"

Fortunately for the forces of reason, or at least machine politics, other foes of Brinkley were more quietly at work. Investigators (whether for Woodring or Landon isn't clear) found his old partner-in-crime James Crawford selling cars in Kansas City, Missouri. They offered him $250 a month to trail along behind Brinkley's campaign and give a speech after every one of his, like a second dog whizzing on a tree. Crawford refused. He had been duped two years before, he said, by a private detective hired by Fishbein's attorneys before Brinkley dropped his suit. Crawford was doing time for armed robbery then—one-armed robbery of a hotel—and he claimed the investigator, named McCoy, had promised to spring him from prison in return for damaging information about the doctor. Crawford supplied some, he said, and got nothing in return but some candy and a box of cigars. He was through helping the AMA.

Sally Wike was busy, however, giving bathetic interviews in an effort to wreck her ex-husband's chances. "The children and myself would have enjoyed a little car of some kind," she said, "and even asked him, John R. Brinkley, for the price, but NO . . ." Her principal champion was a scandal sheet called the *Pink Rag,* whose editorial position was that Brinkley "has a record that would make a sewer throw up." The doctor hired a private eye who trailed her fruitlessly for weeks.

Meanwhile, Norman Baker was being a huge nuisance. Fresh from starting his copycat border blaster in Mexico, he continued his primal struggle for the quack throne by running for governor of Iowa. He hadn't a prayer of winning (in the end he got just five thousand votes), but it gave him the chance to tour his state in a lavender roadster with bulletproof windows and to torment Brinkley with their guaranteed pairing in the public mind.

But the worst damage came from an unexpected source. The bespectacled Alf Landon had been derided early on for having "the charisma of a chemistry professor," but as the campaign wore on, voters began to wonder if this was so bad. Maybe an extreme leader in extreme times wasn't wise after all. Landon seized on this shift, applying himself to the electorate like a warm compress, a paragon of negative virtues:

> He is not a dangerous man to have in the governor's chair. . . .
> Labor will have no cause to be alarmed with Landon in office. . . . Hokum and bunk will have no place in the state house with Landon as governor.

Brinkley lost by more than thirty thousand votes. For all his folksy rhetoric, the doctor never gained the faith of desperate farmers because he never spelled out exactly how he would help them. The Sally factor hurt him with women. Some said that the "implied respectability of major parties" in a presidential-election year was enough to tip the scales.

Desolate and bitter, Brinkley railed at man and God. His black despair brought this reproof from Alma Graning, head of the School of Divine Science and Philosophy in Los Angeles: "You must not reach the conclusion that this thing about a 'hereafter' is 'all the bunk'! Your intelligence does not confirm this thought and it is only the repressing influence of Saturn that makes you feel like this."

On Christmas Eve he turned once more to his greatest consolation. "My Dear Sweetheart," he wrote.

> Do you realize that within another seven months you and I will have been together for twenty years? . . . I have loved you since the first time I ever saw you. . . .

I have no more idea than a man in the moon what the future holds in store for us. . . . Personally I would like to discontinue every business project that I am in and shake loose of the whole mess and start life all over again on a different pathway. However, I have so many obligations to meet so many ways that it seems almost a hopeless thought to try to break loose. . . .

I want you to know that I love you and the baby, and that everything that I do in the way of work or progress is for the good of both of you, and as this Christmas comes to us in 1932, I express to you and my darling boy all my love and I know that you reciprocate every bit of it.

Devotedly yours,
J. R. Brinkley, M.D.

37

By the early 1930s glands and public relations, two of the great fascinations of the day, had penetrated the international scene at the highest levels. Witness the dark machinations of Germany's newest political party. . . .

Back in New York from Berlin, Hearst foreign correspondent Karl von Weigand met with PR wizard Edward Bernays. Over dinner the reporter described to him Joseph Goebbels, one of Hitler's top lieutenants. Bit of an eyesore, Goebbels. Diminutive, with a club foot—hardly your picture-perfect Nazi—and still he had women coming down the chimney. Some called him "the he-goat of Babelsberg." The point was, Goebbels had given a tour of his vast propaganda library, during which he mentioned that he was using Bernays's book *Crystallizing Public Opinion* as a foundation for his campaign against the Jews.

"This shocked me," Bernays later wrote.

Perhaps on reflection Bernays was less shocked than shocked, shocked to discover that while he had been teaching how to manipulate the masses "without their knowing it" to clients like CBS, General Electric, the American Tobacco Company, and Dodge Motors, the Nazis had quietly joined the queue. "Publicity as an instrument of control," how to exploit symbols and hoodwink the press: themes like these were meat and drink to Goebbels, the "Mahatma Propagandhi" of the Third Reich and driving force behind the "Big Lie." Like bestselling author Bruce Barton, Goebbels liked to cite Jesus

Christ as a consummate salesman. "The propagandist," the Nazi said, "must be the man with the greatest knowledge of souls."

But Bernays's work was not the only new science the Third Reich had turned to its own purposes. Inevitably the research of a certain Russian had also captured its fancy:

"The mother who is the first to hand me her child for a rejuvenation operation perhaps would be the founder of a new and mighty human race. . . . Give me children endowed with the spark of genius and I will breed a new race of supermen."

So said Dr. Serge Voronoff in the late 1920s, and when the Nazis came to power they remembered it. When Hitler stood in Munich to proclaim the emergence of the German people from an "ice period of senility," when he declared the need to bring "the physical rejuvenation of the Third Reich into consonance with [its] spiritual resurgence," he wasn't just talking about new gymnasiums.

As rejuvenators the Nazis brought their own ideas to the table. One of their methods for constructing a race of supermen (even better than the naturally occurring Nordic kind) was their involuntary plastic surgery program, whereby the state was authorized to resculpt a soldier's body "against his will if necessary, as to extract from it its maximum fitness." As for Voronoff's work, it's unclear how deeply they explored it—the thought of creating a master race with monkey parts would likely cause cognitive dissonance in most Nazis—but his theories were tested. Steinach's vasectomy method, never. Hitler razed the Austrian's laboratory in 1933, partly because he was a Jew and partly because of his efforts to "cure" homosexuality by transplanting heterosexual testicles into "effeminate, passive" men. In this area the Führer preferred murder to research.

In any case, it didn't take long for German scientists to see more quickly than some that gland transplants were a dead end. But they had caught rejuvenation fever, and they forged ahead with tests of their own. Not all bore fruit. A professor at the Kaiser-Wilhelm-Institut in Mulheim prematurely announced that man could grow younger by eating coal. Soon, however, German investigators gained a cloudy but partially accurate sense of the next frontier. In the fall of 1933 the *New York Times* offered this intriguing glimpse of Nazi efforts to catch youth in a bottle:

German Laboratory Denies Gas Charge

Berlin, Oct 24—To refute charges made by newspapers and periodicals in Great Britain and other countries that the Schering-Kahlbaum company of Berlin was "one of Germany's secret arsenals" manufacturing poison gas, the company, which is one of Germany's biggest chemical and pharmaceutical concerns, opened its laboratory and factory for inspection today by foreign press correspondents. . . .

So far as a layman could observe there was no manufacture of poison gas. It was observed, however, that the concern was spending millions of marks in experiments to isolate the male hormone [testosterone] that is to replace the rejuvenation means of Steinach and Voronoff and is to restore or increase manly vigor and courage. Berlin's policemen were used as subjects.

Animal and clinical experiments, it was said, have already shown good results; they have produced so far no genuine rejuvenation, but have contributed to the restoration of general well-being. . . .

In Del Rio, John Brinkley had shaken off the blues. Not because his spirit had been fired by the Nazis—that would come later—but rather because his lust for cash and zest for invention never deserted him for long.

He was making lemonade from the lemons of '32. That idea he'd had about a sound truck delivering prerecorded speeches—he now adapted it to the music business. Live sets on XER were mixed with sets "recorded live" on sixteen-inch disks chiseled with a Presto transcription cutter. At first Brinkley used them early in the morning so performers could sleep late, but the broader potential of "electrical transcription" was instantly apparent, both for music and the spoken word. The prerecorded commercial was born. For the doctor it didn't come a moment too soon; around this same time Congress passed a law aimed directly at him. He was still giving some radio talks in Milford and sending them south by telephone to his Mexican transmitter. The new legislation carried a "Brinkley clause" that banned this technique. His response was to slap his voice onto records and ship them across the border. The mouse stayed a step ahead of the cat.

For those who practiced to deceive, transcription was a garden of opportunity. Brinkley at once took advantage. Of the local artists he employed, soprano Rosa Dominguez, aka "Mexico's Nightingale," was the best-loved. Unfortunately Lydia Mendoza, "the Lark of the Border," was even more popular, and she worked at a rival station. One day she began to work for Brinkley, too. She sang over XER, she chatted with the announcer. . . .

"They used to say that I was there in person in the studio during the broadcast," the Lark of the Border later wrote, "that I was singing live. And they would ask, 'Lydia Mendoza, which song are you going to sing?' and things like that. . . . [S]omeone took on the role of being me, so that they could pretend that I was actually there." Mendoza hired a lawyer who threatened to sue unless Brinkley desisted. He did, though he continued to sell "autographed photos" of her for a dollar apiece.

In late summer he decided to consolidate his interests. Barred from practicing medicine in Kansas and twice beaten for the governorship, Brinkley closed his hospital there and opened a new one in Del Rio, on three floors of the Roswell Hotel. On October 7, 1933, he and Minnie left Milford for the last time at the head of a modern wagon train: thirty radio and hospital personnel and their families. Along with them went every stick of furniture, all the equipment, every chandelier and sconce Brinkley had been able to rip out before bringing in the wrecking ball. The only thing he left behind was a massive pile of debris.

Del Rio didn't just welcome Brinkley; it practically hugged him around the knees. The town stood to gain even more from the new hospital than it had from XER, starting with a $20,000-a-week payroll juicing the local economy. All those patients streaming in translated into more tourists than the new "Dollar Rio" knew what to do with. In the evenings folks danced to live music in the park. Ma Crosby's café was packed. Even Boys' Town, the red-light district across the bridge, got a major upgrade thanks to all the men heading there to try out their new glands. "[Brinkley] has an arresting and highly magnetic radio personality which radiates confidence, faith and sincerity," an American diplomat wrote glumly to Secretary of State Cordell Hull. "There is great enthusiasm in the town for him and apparently everyone is happy except the doctors."

To lure more trade, Brinkley talked up the region's charms on the radio. He rhapsodized over Del Rio's delightful jumble of cultures, the burros threading among the automobiles, the health-giving pools at San Felipe Springs, the Texas sunsets "as glorious as those that kiss the bounding billows of the Mediterranean into a flame of gold." North of town were ranches where they raised goats. It was kismet. "Come visit us," the doctor said, "where summer spends the winter," perhaps lifting a line from the Arizona Chamber of Commerce.

Meanwhile, Milford and Sally Wike had a lot in common.

A Bitter Milford Now

The Kansas Town Turns on Brinkley in Wrath

Yellow Paint Is Smeared on One of His Signs and His Name Is Chiseled from a Building by the Citizens of the Community
—*local headlines*, December 7, 1933

Not everyone had left. Those two long-trusted lieutenants, Drs. Owensby and Dragoo, chose to stay behind, and just before the boss's departure they had surreptitiously copied his client list. Now they did the very thing that Brinkley, by demolishing his buildings, had hoped to prevent: they set up nearby and went into business for themselves.

When the doctor heard about it, he mailed out fifteen thousand dolorous form letters to names on the pirated list. He and Minnie, he wrote, "are down here in Del Rio, Texas. . . . This is our final move until we move to that last resting place from which none ever return.

"If your heart goes out in sympathy to we two mortals who have suffered so much abuse and lost almost everything we have because we have dared to do something for suffering humanity—then I know your sense of Loyalty will cause you to support Dr. and Mrs. Brinkley and not those who have betrayed our confidence."

38

By now there was a fair-sized school of thought that Fishbein's cure—running Brinkley out of Kansas—had been worse than the disease, given the present power of XER and its alien spawn. Fishbein could hardly deny it himself as complaints and appeals piled up on his desk:

> "I received absolutely no relief from the operation. . . . I think Dr. Brinkley and his associates are the biggest bunch of swindlers I ever met."

> "I am writing this letter because I feel that the men should know what a fake he is . . ."

> "I was one of Dr. Brinkley's victims to the tune of $600 . . ."

But with the doctor set up safely across the border, Fishbein could no more get at him than a dog prowling back and forth behind a locked gate. When *JAMA* attacked him, Brinkley fleeringly told his listeners not to be "deranged by the psycho-bunko" of Fishy Fishbein's vendetta, and went on vacuuming in corners for every possible nickel: "I know you are hard up for money. We are too. If you have some farm land, city property, stocks, bonds or other property that may have some value in the future but upon which you cannot realize money now and are sick and in need, write me what you have and we will help you if we can."

Fishbein still had allies in America's broadcasting networks (NBC and CBS) and the State Department, all as eager as he was to put the blasters out of business. Now promising justice at last, that is, a better sharing of bandwidths, American diplomats persuaded Mexico to host a North American Radio Conference in July of 1933. That it was planned as a necktie party for the doctor was obvious to all, including Brinkley himself, who sent a squad of sixteen lawyers and public relations operatives to defend his interests.

Charley Curtis himself led this delegation. As Fishbein's minions reportedly "lurked in the shadows," the former vice president lauded his client as the greatest physician in the hemisphere and declared that Brinkley's work with goats was a sensational achievement. If "Senator [Thomas] Sterling of South Dakota and two or three others in the seats of the almighty had gone to Dr. Brinkley's hospital for treatment," Curtis said, "they would now be alive." In the end his bluster and bravado were sufficient (and America's offers to Mexico insufficient) to carry the day. The conference collapsed, leaving Brinkley still in place.

But his throne was never safe. In early 1934 fickle Mexico changed its mind once more and announced it was shutting down XER. Unceasing pressure from America was a factor, but the decision came mostly from within. Ever since Brinkley's reign began, Mexico had suffered stabs of buyer's remorse. Officials, and the country as a whole, could never seem to decide whether his presence was a blot or a plus, and either way the aggravation was ceaseless. When the president decided to close him down, even Minnie's last-minute trip to the capital with a satchel full of cash couldn't prevent it.

Again Fishbein dared to hope.

On February 24, 1934, soldiers arrived in Villa Acuna to seize the station. According to one report "a violent confrontation was narrowly avoided between the federal troops and local citizenry loyal to the doctor," with the Villa Acuna police, who liked the uniforms he'd bought them, ready to join the resistance. But Brinkley, in another passion-play moment, intervened. He would sacrifice the station temporarily, he said, to avoid bloodshed. "I desire an amicable settlement with the Mexican government," he told his radio audience next day. "In closing the largest, most powerful broadcasting station in the world, the Mexican people will suffer. . . . But I shall be back with you again, my dear, dear friends."

He promptly sued the Mexican government for breach of contract, then went right back on the air through a patchwork of other stations north and south of the Rio Grande. From February 1934 to November 1935, via telephone lines and recordings, he broadcast night and day from Colorado, Kansas, and Missouri. He bought a small border blaster, XEPN at Piedras Negras, began expanding that, then acquired XEAW at Reynosa, too. The authorities couldn't keep up.

His mass mailings grew more elaborate and more aggressive than ever. Anyone who replied, however idly, to one of his flyers was peppered with finely tuned follow-ups. Their tone was pleasant the first two or three times. Then . . .

Fourth Follow-up:

Is the joke on me?

Your request for more literature led me to believe you were intending to come and see me and I sent it gladly.

You have not made an appointment and I'm wondering if you were just "kidding" me. . . . If you have no intentions of coming to see me just say so and there will be no hard feelings.

Honesty is always the best policy.

Fifth Follow-up:

Just what kind of a fellow are you?

You wrote to us for information regarding our work and we sent it to you. . . . Now after we have sent you literature and have written you . . . we can't even hear from you.

Sixth Follow-up:

The above is final notice. . . . Do not ask for one second's extension. It will not be granted.

And as the recipient trudged back from his mailbox into the house, opening yet another envelope, there was that voice again on the radio twanging like a two-string guitar:

"I've found that when folks are restored to normal sexual strength they have an entirely different view of life. It becomes sweet to them again. But take a man, castrate him, and he begins to revert to the feminine. His voice cracks, his beard disappears, his hips round and his breasts enlarge . . ."

The system wasn't perfect. After one E. E. Cooper died of blood poisoning at Brinkley's hospital, a letter arrived at his home inviting him to tour the premises. His widow raised a tremendous stink.

After twenty months, Mexico's highest court ruled that the government had breached its contract with Brinkley and illegally seized his station. Rechristened XERA, it returned to the air December 1, with the doctor back in the catbird seat.

"My dear friends, my patients, my supplicants," he intoned. "Your many, many letters—many hundreds of them since yesterday— lie here before me, touching testimony of your pain, your grief, the wretchedness that is visited upon the innocent."

Growing portly now, hair receding, "the most learned doctor in America" would take in $12 million during the worst years of the Depression—a time when the average general practitioner in the United States earned $3,000 to $3,500 annually and a specialist less than $7,000. Spreading cash across twenty bank accounts in five states, he invested in timber, citrus groves, and real estate, including seven thousand acres in North Carolina near his boyhood home. And he did it all, or nearly all, without goats.

Not long after shifting his practice to Del Rio, Brinkley made the stupendous announcement that he was giving up goat-gland transplants. He had devised a new surgery for boosting sex drive, he said, a simpler procedure capable of effecting "a change of relationship between the epididymus and the gland itself." What this meant— well, what difference did it make? "The results are astounding. I can say truthfully that keeping in almost weekly touch with the some 700 patients that I have operated on here in Del Rio, Texas, that I am producing 100% results."

He dubbed this new technique—in a rare nod to a competitor— "Steinach No. 2," while stressing that the turbine thus produced far outstripped Steinach No. 1. In truth, all Brinkley added to the standard vasectomy was a squirt of Mercurochrome, which caused the customer to emit colored urine for a couple of days: ocular proof of big science. Asked how long its effects would last, Mrs. Brinkley replied tartly, "Till Gabriel blows his trumpet on Judgment Day, and then they'll have to knock you on the head with a mallet." Of course, if the patient was rich enough and absolutely insisted, Brinkley could still dig up a goat somewhere. Huey Long reportedly made an appointment to get goat glands in Del Rio but was assassinated before he could get there.

Primarily, though, it was that beautiful bottleneck, the prostate, that was Brinkley's pet now, the "star of the literature" he mailed to prospective clients. There were at least thirty-six million American males out there over forty, and a lot of them who thought rejuvenation too zany still had to cope with "the old cocklebur." "You know your prostate's infected and diseased. . . . Why do you twist and squirm around . . . when I am offering you these low rates, this easy work, this lifetime-of-service plan? Come at once to the Brinkley Hospital before it is everlastingly too late."

Even younger men, Brinkley said, especially those who had been all too quick "to offer their bodies on the Altar of Eros," should hurry in for a checkup. Again he drew a veil over the trade-secret details: "Not even Mrs. Brinkley knows my secret," he said. But he assured the world that the technique would make his name "stand out in bold relief among the great luminaries of this generation," while annihilating pretenders like the Prostate Gland Warmer, complete with blue lightbulb ("stimulate the abdominal brain!"), and the Recto Rotor, a device every bit as alarming as its name implied.

Brinkley's prostate-softening plan came in three varieties: Poor

Folks' ($150), Average Man's ($750), and Business Man's ($1,000). The last was recommended for owners of "the finest automobiles, the finest homes, the best horses, best diamonds, best works of art," and promised the "Compound Technique, the 'Rock of Gibraltar' of Dr. Brinkley's work." After surgery, each patient was charged an extra $100 for six tiny bottles of Formula 1020, to be injected sequentially once he got back home.

"What more do you want, folks?"

How about a second hospital in San Juan, Texas, this one specializing in "diseases of the female and male rectum"? And, ladies, while you're there, "Don't forget the estrogens we are now able to give you for loss of sexual strength. . . . Wonderful sexual strength may be returned.

"Remember, Del Rio for the prostate and San Juan for the colon!"

The log-cabin baby had grown into an empire builder. A saga like that belonged between hard covers, and in the mid-1930s Brinkley hired a struggling poet named Clement Wood to write it for him. The result of their collaboration was *Life of a Man* and its leitmotif was no surprise: ". . . that criticism which crucified Jesus Christ, stoned Stephen, hooted Paul for a madman, tried Luther for a criminal, tortured Galileo, bound Columbus in chains, drove Dante into the hell of exile . . . of their company is John R. Brinkley." Amid moist paeans to this man who "could not be bound by the rigid, artificial ethics of the American Medical Association" there was this striking passage, a where-are-they-now inventory of the members of the Kansas State Medical Board who had revoked his license there in 1930:

Dr. Jenkins . . . was instantly killed, and horribly mangled, limb from limb, by a railroad train. Dr. Hissem, another member, died, it was said, from a broken heart, following the death of his only son, a prominent Wichita surgeon, whose automobile ran into a cement bridge. Dr. Ross, another member, lost his wife soon after the revocation of Brinkley's license. Brinkley was told that he lost his mind from grieving over this loss, and, some said, over his injustice to

Brinkley; that neighbors found him walking around dressed in his wife's clothes, and had to take care of him. . . .

Do not think that Brinkley did not observe all this, with a sad serene relish. He is a philosopher, as well as so much else; and he is a devout believer in divine justice. . . . [He] has noticed, with a queer inner satisfaction, that no individual, no group, no organization, that has ever fought against him, has failed to meet with disaster.

Around the same time Brinkley made a promotional film that toured theaters across the country. It opens like a Robert Benchley short, with the doctor sitting at his desk.

"Hello, my friends in Texas, Kansas and everywhere. This is Dr. Brinkley speaking to you from my lovely home in Del Rio, Texas, where summer spends the winter."

For a couple of minutes he delivers his million-dollar mixture of the down-home and the incomprehensible. Then in a tone of wooden surprise: "Oh, look who's here." Minnie crosses to him, pecks him on the cheek, and says to the camera: "You'd better listen to Doctor, or you'll be much worse off than you are now. . . . But excuse me, I have to go off to the kitchen to cook our Sunday dinner." Brinkley gazes after her, then turns to the audience: "You can trust what Minnie says, folks. After all, she just came from communion."

39

If I owned Hell and Texas," Union General Philip Sheridan once said, "I'd live in Hell and rent out Texas." That remark may or may not have been confined to the weather, but true it was that by June, Del Rio was hotter than two goats in a pepper patch, and a man of Brinkley's resources wasn't about to stick around for it. Instead, each summer he, Minnie, and Johnny Boy set forth on an exotic three-month vacation. Much of that time they spent at sea, for as a Detroit paper noted in March 1934, "the loquacious purveyor of goat giblets has bought a yacht."

In fact there were three yachts in succession, the *Dr. Brinkley I,* the *Dr. Brinkley II,* and the *Dr. Brinkley III.* The last and largest was 172 feet long and carried a crew of twenty-one. All wore identical shirts embroidered with the doctor's name, while he himself strode the deck in an admiral's uniform complete with gold buttons and a sword. "[W]e just had a wonderful life," Minnie recalled. "We traveled both Atlantic and Pacific oceans, and to the South Seas, Central America and South America on the Pacific side." In the South Pacific they feasted on turtles' eggs and paid a visit to Devil's Island, a trip Johnny Boy later wrote about for school: "A trusty who killed three women showed us the shops where shoes, clothing and furniture were made. We had cocoa, nut milk and pineapple crush, served by the warden at this office. There we saw a monkey hanging by its tail; and upon inquiry found out the monkey belonged to a criminal, who sold it to daddy." The admiral also came away with a parrot and a mahogany walking cane.

In Nassau, a favorite port of call, the Brinkleys became friends with the Duke and Duchess of Windsor (the former King Edward VIII and Wallis Simpson), whose recent marriage Mencken had called "the greatest news story since the Resurrection." Minnie said, "I'd go out to the country club in the afternoon—they had a box there—and I'd sit in the box with the duchess while the duke played polo." One year the doctor rented them his yacht.

Sport fishing was his great passion. There was no humbug about it: Brinkley had a thirst for adventure, and in battling a marlin or big tuna he could have gone toe to toe with Hemingway. In the summer of 1935 he and his family, accompanied by chief aide Dr. Osborn and his wife, cruised up the eastern coast of the United States, headed toward tuna season in the north Atlantic. After taking in the Harvard-Yale crewing races off Connecticut, they continued on toward Canada. On June 30 they ran aground.

In dense fog off Nova Scotia, the yacht had been sucked ashore by the current near the Bay of Fundy. Everyone aboard was safely rescued, and damage to the vessel was not severe. The Brinkleys got to meet some locals. ("We're simple people," the doctor said, "easy as an old shoe. Even in an admiral's uniform I don't get all swelled up.") A private motor launch was hired to refloat it, and soon the yacht was back on course.

In Halifax the ship was seized and Brinkley arrested for skipping out on the bill for his salvage, but he settled up and was on his way.

Long days followed on the open sea, riding the heave and slap of the water. They reached Liverpool, Nova Scotia, on August 8 and anchored in a grove of schooners and small craft. The timing was excellent. In mid-August masses of herring made their annual Pamplona-style rush through these waters with hungry tuna in pursuit: blue torpedoes that skimmed up almost to the surface, then reangled and vanished. The doctor hired a couple of local salts to help him, and they set out before dawn on August 10.

He hooked one that same day. He fought it for hours, the full fifteen rounds, till finally the exhausted fish rolled up alongside the boat where it was gaffed and dragged aboard. It weighed 690 pounds—according to the *New York Times,* "the largest caught in Atlantic waters this season." Later the doctor had it stuffed, mounted, and presented to the Del Rio high school.

An excellent trophy, but it paled beside one he landed after that. At 788 pounds, it surpassed the record held by Western novelist Zane Grey. It was, up to that time, the largest tuna ever caught in the western hemisphere.

40

But O that I were young again
And held her in my arms.

— WILLIAM BUTLER YEATS

Ten years after the runaway success of *Black Oxen,* the saga of the rejuvenated Madame Zattiany, Gertrude Atherton was promoting her latest novel, written from the point of view of an eighteen-year-old niece of the poet Horace. Speaking to an audience in San Francisco, the acclaimed authoress, now seventy-eight, was dressed in a black satin gown with a pink satin jacket trimmed in feathers, her nails and lips carmined, her hair in a golden pompadour. She said she had ovarian radiation to thank for the ease with which she had channeled a Roman teenager, a creation "so real that she seemed to be doing the writing."

Asked to comment on Miss Atherton's speech, Morris Fishbein mildly replied that the benefits claimed were "largely in the effect on the mind of the patient."

Nearly twenty years on, Fishbein and his allies must have been wondering if the madness would ever end. William Butler Yeats, considered by many the greatest poet of the age, had just been Steinached at the age of sixty-nine. The "strange second puberty" he felt afterward carried him into an affair with a twenty-seven-year-old actress. Steinach himself, though still snarling at the press for distorting his work, continued to promise that "the process of getting old can be reversed." Dr. Serge Voronoff—now on his third wife, a twenty-year-old Austrian belle—touted monkey glands as eagerly as ever, though proof, like prosperity, was always just around the corner.

Then in the fall of 1935 came the breakthrough several scientists had been groping toward: Swiss chemist Leopold Ruzicka and Adolph Butenandt of Germany, working independently, isolated and manufactured the male hormone, testosterone. As *Time* magazine explained, there was great hope now that this feat would "put to the test the rejuvenation theories that came into prominence with the monkey and goat gland sensations," or even supersede them altogether. Perhaps as the Nazis had posited, testosterone was the magic key to the land of lost time. And if that was true, there must be a parallel doorway for women. Instead of enduring surgery, people might someday reverse the aging process with simple injections—or even pills, like dieters ("I lost fifteen years in three weeks!").

At fifty-six, H. L. Mencken was feeling his age. It was not fading sexual strength that worried him so much as loss of mental potency, his zest for life. The Great Skeptic feared that his prodigious energy for work might be draining away.

In December 1936 he checked into Johns Hopkins Hospital with yet another ragbag of complaints. His medical file listed them as: "Tickling in back of throat, present for six days, with malaise, muscle pains and very mild fever. Diagnosis: Acute infectional tracheitis; acute infectional sinusitis; acute epididymitis (right) cause unknown."

During his stay at Johns Hopkins he underwent two significant treatments. First "a cyst was removed from the right epididymus." Then he was wheeled into the operating room, where he was quietly and improbably Steinached.

41

When President Franklin Roosevelt ran for reelection in 1936, his Republican opponent was the governor of Kansas. Alf Landon even wore a sunflower in his lapel, just as Brinkley used to do. For the doctor, the presidential campaign that autumn was a long, cruel might-have-been.

On the other hand, he had achieved his original dream: he was richer than a crème brûlée. Wallowing in wealth brought a thousand consolations. Rarely, in fact, does a man so fantastically calculating in acquiring money spend it with such abandon, straight from the id.

On a trip to New York City in the early 1920s he bought Minnie ropes of jewels, a fur coat, and a Stutz Bearcat. That signaled the start of a spending spree that would last nearly two decades. It peaked in Del Rio, where he bought himself a herd of a dozen Cadillacs, but the cars were just a detail. It was the home he created there—a mission-style manor and grounds near the Rio Grande—that had Texas talking: sixteen acres of naked self-regard, part Versailles, part Barnum & Bailey.

His driveway was Del Rio's widest boulevard. Lined with imported palm trees and five-globe streetlights that burned through the night, it led to towering wrought-iron gates crowned with Brinkley's name. Behind the grillwork lay an isle of lush, close-cropped Bermuda grass—"sort of a giant golf course fairway," a visitor said, "dropped in the middle of sagebrush." To the novelty of grass he added a fountain pool adorned with water lilies, a greenhouse (aka "Just a Little Bit of Heaven"), an eight-thousand-bush garden foaming with roses and a wandering zoo: geese, peacocks, celery-chewing tortoises kidnapped from the Galápagos Islands, a couple of flamingos, and a flock of penguins tottering about as if delirious from the heat. More palm trees, each nourished by a buried four-hundred-pound block of ice, ringed a jumbo swimming pool with underwater lighting and a ten-foot diving tower. In the parti-colored tile surrounding the pool, BRINKLEY was rendered three times in mosaic.

At night the grounds were a fairyland. People came from far and wide just to sit in their cars outside the gates and watch the fountains shoot skyward thirty-foot parabolas of water, while beams of light played on them in a dozen ever-changing colors.

Gratifying as all this must have been to the man whose name appeared in flashing neon over the pool between reproductions of classical sculpture, it did have its drawbacks. "How he would fret," Minnie Brinkley remembered, "when he would drive in and have to wait while three-hundred-pound tortoises slowly crossed the driveway." When at last he achieved the door, however, she and a squad of servants were there to welcome him home from the wars. His collection of Italian mirrors loyally repeated his reflection down the hall. Persian rugs, Swiss grandfather clocks, ebony elephants, chess sets, statuary of Carrara marble and bronze: spectacular keepsakes of the Brinkleys' summer voyages crowded fourteen rooms. One guest described the doctor as living "in the style of an Austrian Archduke," but that suggests conceptual coherence. If there was any unifying theme here, it was acquisition itself.

The living room was where he relaxed. After dark, chandeliers of Czechoslovakian crystal flattered some 2,400 square feet of treasures, the largest of which was a cathedral-style, state-of-the-art pipe organ rising two stories high. (No musician, Brinkley hired away the organist at Grauman's Chinese Theater in Hollywood to play it for him.) Other loot included a rosewood piano once owned by film star Norma Talmadge, a six-hundred-year-old tapestry presented to him by the Chinese government, cases of cut-glass crystal with BRINKLEY etched on each piece, an international collection of perfumes, and oversized wall photos of the master of the house. The most striking of these, four feet high and hand colored, showed Brinkley in full admiral's uniform standing beside his record-breaking catch; it was entitled *Tuna Fish and Self.* An art deco marble staircase swooped upward to circular bedrooms of bird's-eye maple and bathrooms in red and deep purple.

As Brinkley liked to say, "For a poor boy, up from bare feet in Jackson County, North Carolina, this, dog me, is something." But at least one visitor, a Del Rio resident named Zina Worley, came away sobered by what she saw. To an out-of-state friend she wrote: "He was completely lacking in any education outside his own field I should think judging by his ostentation, his absence of good taste. Obviously he was eaten with vanity and ambition and his only measure of success was in terms of dollars and influence. . . . It must be a terrible thing to have to keep telling the world how great you are and to want so badly to achieve what is really impossible. We have much to fear from these people, but in a sense, I think, they are tragic."

At least twice Brinkley had the exterior of the mansion repainted—red, then apple green—and his Cadillacs repainted to match. Each Christmas he and Minnie distributed food baskets to the poor. His generous financial contributions earned him the gratitude and friendship of J. Andrew Arnett, head of the Texas Society for the Friendless, and Father Flanagan of Boys' Town.

The doctor was elected president of the Del Rio Rotary Club.

42

In April 1937, while a stunt pilot did barrel rolls in the opalescent evening sky, fourteen hundred guests milled about the Brinkley estate under a wide web of glowing paper lanterns. Floodlights buried in the bushes produced an effect of "intense moonlight, almost as bright as day, such as seen in Japan in the cherry blossom time." High-school girls dressed as geishas hoisted seventy pounds of canapés. From a twinkling bandstand a San Antonio hotel orchestra dealt out dance music and the blues.

It was the biggest party the doctor ever threw, the biggest south Texas could recall. After short speeches and a big feed, the night was crowned by an apocalyptic fireworks display: dogs, cats, ducks, soldiers on horseback appeared in the heavens etched in flame, each greeted with gasps and applause. The last rocket spelled a message that shimmered and flared among the stars:

BON VOYAGE DR MRS BRINKLEY AND JOHNNIE

In mid-June, after giving himself this affectionate send-off, the doctor took his family and, along with the boy's tutor, embarked for Europe aboard the *Queen Mary*. The international Rotary Club convention was in Nice that year, and the doctor was to represent Del Rio. Pulling out of New York harbor, he just missed the new issue of *Time* magazine with Morris Fishbein on the cover.

It had been a difficult spring for Dr. Fishbein. A bad cold had given way to an attack of Bell's palsy, which had the unsettling effect of leaving one side of his face hanging "as slack as a bloodhound's jowls." He made light of it in *JAMA:* "It seems strange to see one side of the countenance so cold and fishy. Belike it would be well to save this appearance to bestow upon the quacks." But the treatment was no joke: doctors strapped his head into a brace for three weeks, forcing the muscles up, and applied electric currents. What separated the quackish from the cutting-edge in this case is obscure, but Fishbein accepted it without complaint. "I am not suffering pain or illness," he wrote Paul DeKruif, "except to the extent that my appearance and the motility of my face are depreciated."

Still, having his picture (sans palsy) on the cover of *Time* gave his spirits a welcome boost, especially since the magazine portrayed him not only as the face of organized medicine but as the Atlas holding it up. "Upon the *Journal* which Dr. Fishbein edits the AMA depends for practically every dollar of its operating expenses," the article reported, and offered figures to prove it. There was little mention of the enemies he'd made, especially the pockets of resentment in-house—the doctors who didn't like his trumpeting personal opinions as if he were speaking ex cathedra; the pesky minority who thought he was too conservative. There was no word of the Chicago Medical Society's attempt to have him disciplined when he dismissed innovations in obstetrics as "fads and frills."

Yet he couldn't have done without his enemies, those within the AMA and without. To him and Brinkley both, the unopposed life was not worth living. In that sense they were made for each other.

Both stood in 1937 at the apex of their careers. Both went to Europe that summer. Both took their families along.

Following a physicians' convention in Belfast, the Fishbeins planned a tour of Scandinavia.

When the *Queen Mary* docked in Cherbourg on May 31, a chauffeured limousine swallowed the Brinkleys at the pier and bore them south to the Mediterranean. This wasn't the first time Rotary Clubbers had picked Nice as their place to play. Along with the beauty of the setting, there was just enough gunfire, knife play, and drunken driving—the previous year a traffic cop had been hospitalized seven times—to make for a bracing holiday. There were even reports of a band of swindlers dressed as priests.

After the convention the Brinkleys did the full grand tour, a glittering ten-week sweep of Paris, Dijon, Grenoble, Cannes; Rome, Naples, Florence, Venice; Yugoslavia, Belgium, Luxembourg, and the United Kingdom. There was gratifying fanfare along the way: in Dublin, for instance, they were feted by the Lord Mayor. But the doctor's favorite stop was Berlin, where at last he could see the Third Reich up close.

Had he arrived in the city just a couple of years before, he would have found filth, dilapidation, and citizens guarding their potatoes with guns; once Berlin was tapped for the 1936 Olympics, however, Hitler broke out the buckets and brooms, and now even the cobblestones between the trolley tracks were clean as a whistle. Columns of soldiers boot-slapped down every boulevard; "Hitler's cross" hung everywhere; there were loudspeakers in the trees. These were people, Brinkley saw, who understood the science of worship.

At last, laden with souvenirs, the family departed Europe for home on August 11, 1937, putting out from Southampton, England, in a heavy fog. This time they were booked on the fabled French ship the *Normandie*.

In the Depression-defying rage for luxury liners, the *Normandie* was the ne plus ultra: the most spectacular and the most sumptuous, the first to exceed one thousand feet in length—making it, a New York reporter decided, "3½ times bigger" than Noah's Ark. By any measure the *Normandie* beat a boatful of animals. From its grand lounge (a colossal crystal box with panoramic bas-reliefs) to its Ottoman Empire chapel with geometric Christ to its smoking room, a forest of etched-glass murals and lustrous panels on Egyptian, Greek, and Japanese themes, the Ship of Light boggled even the most blasé. The dining room for first-class passengers—"a miraculous grotto, an Ali Baba cave"—was longer than the Hall of Mirrors at Versailles and starred the most sophisticated French cuisine. British diplomat Harold Nicholson wrote to his wife, Vita Sackville-West: "I have never known such luxury . . . it would drive me mad after a week." Brinkley, made of sterner stuff, reportedly took the best suite onboard. If so, he was living better than King Tut died.

For those who could stop gawking there was lots to do. During the four-day voyage Johnny Boy's tutor, Lowell Brown, wrote he was "well entertained with picture shows, dancing, fine swimming pool, dummy horse races, ping pong, boxing and fencing exhibitions." After the boxing matches—Henry Fonda was a popular guest referee— there was always a pillow fight: six blindfolded pages flailing away at each other while the crowd howled.

Best of all, Brown started up a shipboard romance with an effervescent physician's daughter, seventeen years old. With the rest of her family she, too, was returning home from a long European jaunt. The young tutor and the girl played Ping-Pong, then drifted on deck, where down the way tweedy gentlemen fired helplessly at clay pigeons in the whipping breeze. The sting of the sea, the far horizon, the massive ship carving the waves: in a setting like this flirtation rises to the level of epic poetry. By next day the pair had graduated to hitting golf balls into a net, the perfect chance for a young man to help his new friend adjust her swing.

His tutor's romancing gave Johnny Boy a rare chance to slip the leash. The ten-year-old was growing moodier with each passing year. Since the age of three he had been a quack in training, adorably reading listener letters on the air after drilling on words like *hemorrhoids* and *tonsillectomy*. He sang "Happy Birthday" to young friends he didn't know. Owner of a green Cadillac he was years away from driving, he walked to school with a bodyguard who clung to him all day and then trailed him home. Other kids mocked him of course. "The doctor worshiped Johnny and denied him nothing," said a childhood friend. "But Johnny was the unhappiest person I've ever known."

Down the corridors of the *Normandie* he stole. A stray door might open onto acrobats or magicians—it had happened before, but that was at night. Once or twice he got lost, but then there it was: the children's playroom at the base of the forward smokestack.

It was like stepping into a brilliantly illustrated storybook. The walls were covered with dolls and fairy-tale characters dancing in a rain of musical notes. There were polka-dotted horses on springs to ride, even a Punch and Judy theater. Right now the little stage was curtained and closed. There was no one about.

Johnny was rooting in the toy box when the door opened and another boy came in.

He, too, was ten years old. His family had nicknamed him "the Menace" for the speed with which he went through nannies. But to the little gentleman across the room he introduced himself simply as Justin Fishbein.

They asked each other the usual questions. "What does your father do?" Justin said, digging in the box. "Mine's a doctor."

"My father's a doctor, too," Johnny replied, "but the other doctors don't like him."

This puzzled Justin. It didn't seem fair. Later on he told his father about this nice boy he'd met, a doctor's son, who was down in the mouth about the way other doctors treated his dad. Justin asked if there was anything his father could do about it. Fishbein asked the doctor's name.

Meanwhile it was just a matter of time before Lowell Brown got to chatting with his new flame about his employer. "Do you know who my boss is?" he asked Marjorie Fishbein between golf swings. She didn't, so he told her. "She terminated the conversation rather abruptly," Brown said later. "I think we spoke a time or two after that but never associated any more."

There was nothing left now but for the principals to meet. In all these years, the two great foes had never laid eyes on each other, and Fishbein wanted to keep it that way. Brinkley had other ideas.

Scouring the deck, he found Fishbein in a lounge chair with a book on his chest and his face to the sun. Brinkley approached and stopped a few feet away. The other roused as if from sleep, blinked, and returned to reading his book.

Brinkley came nearer and stopped again. For once he couldn't seem to get a word out. He shifted here and there, as if demonstrating indignation from different angles, while Fishbein pretended he wasn't there. After a minute or so of this queer pantomime, Brinkley made a strangled noise, turned, and stalked off.

Not a word exchanged. What an anticlimax—or so one might have thought. But beholding him, the quack in the flesh, woke something in Fishbein: it whetted his almost blunted purpose. He stepped off the ship in New York resolved to destroy that scoundrel once and for all.

43

Back home in Chicago, Fishbein penned a two-part article, "Modern Medical Charlatans." He threw everything at Brinkley but the kitchen sink. The first installment was scheduled for the January issue of the layman's journal *Hygeia*.

In the meantime the editor was invited to Hollywood, where he underwent an experience familiar to many modern authors: being diddled by a movie studio. What the executives at Warner Brothers had in mind was a two-fisted quackery melodrama—working title *Your Life Is in Their Hands*—based on cases from Fishbein's files. He would serve as technical adviser and, according to Louella Parsons's column, "Paul Muni, who owes Warners one more story, will be invited to play the lead."

When that got out, alternative healers of every stripe erupted. Chiropractors, optometrists, and osteopaths, on whom Fishbein still dumped with regularity, were sure that "anyone who is not an MD will be ridiculed in this picture." The controversy proved too much for Warners, which caved and canceled the project.

Brinkley, too, had returned home filled with a new sense of purpose. Germany had set his mind soaring. Who needed elected office? Political power was his for the taking. Thanks to his radio command post, he was brilliantly positioned for a new role, the ultimate in autointoxication: John Brinkley, right-wing demagogue.

In his idiosyncratic brand of Christianity, a mix of mercenary calculation and confusing himself with the Lord, an anti-Semitic element had always lurked. Campaigning for governor back in 1932, he had earned the endorsement of Reverend Gerald B. Winrod, a Wichita preacher who traced most of the world's ills to an international Jewish conspiracy and all its blessings to "old-fashioned, God-fearing, baby-having Americans." The explosion of European fascism in the desperate thirties had like-minded types in the United States emerging like snakes from a drain. Father Coughlin with his creepy brogue; Fritz Kuhn, "the American Führer"; William D. Pelley, who founded the Silver Shirts the day after the Nazis took power: these were America's best-known hatemongers, and all three after Brinkley's return to Del Rio appeared as guests on XERA. Though he largely agreed with them, and even contributed five thousand dollars to Pelley's cause, the doctor himself was not as explicitly virulent as they. On air, at least, he preferred the role of sentimental isolationist: "War is the Communist's delight. He mixes its bitter broth for the sweet lips of your boy. . . . I would deport every radical who preferred the gleam of warlike Mars to the soft amber light of the Bethlehem orb."

But he added tiny swastikas to the tile around his pool.

Inveighing against the "red menace," fifth columnists, "parlor pink" liberals, and all the rest trying to make Hitler's life harder, he ran little risk of antagonizing customers. Memories of the 1914 to 1918 world war were still fresh, and few of his listeners were eager for a second. That meant supporting isolationism actually helped sell prostate operations and colonic cleansings, just as it helped sell mail-order products that were bogus, ill-made, or potentially fatal.

Brinkley never looked beyond that, so he never understood his real impact. He never saw that it was his entertainment programming—the music streaming out of XERA, intended as a sop, a lure—that had sparked something much bigger: a full-scale cultural upheaval. For years now, while his mind was elsewhere, Brinkley had been offering a free Ph.D. in country and Tex-Mex music to:

... Chet Atkins, a teenager in Columbus, Georgia, who tuned in to XERA on a battery-powered radio he built from mail-order parts

... Waylon Jennings, a youngster in Littlefield, Texas, whose daddy ran a cable from his truck battery into the house so the family could listen to XERA

... Tom T. Hall, future songwriter and balladeer in Olive Hill, Kentucky

... Johnny Cash in Dyess, Arkansas, who first heard his future bride June Carter, then age ten, singing over Brinkley's airwaves

The "Original Carter Family"—A.P., Sara, and Maybelle—first appeared on XERA after Brinkley's return from Europe. When he hired them, the doc knew little about the Carters except that they were popular in the southeast. Discovered by Victor talent scout Ralph Peer a decade earlier, the trio had sold thousands of records regionally: "Worried Man Blues," "Will the Circle Be Unbroken?" and many more. No longer. The Depression had wrecked sales in the hillbilly record business. So, reluctant though they were to leave their little corner of Virginia, when Ralph Peer wangled them a slot on Brinkley's station—two shows a day for six months, seventy-five dollars a week each, six months paid vacation—they took it. The job came with fringe benefits, too, though nobody realized it at the time. Their three-year stint on XERA would turn the Carter Family from regional stars into national icons, "the inventors of commercial country music," "the big bang of country music," the first act elected to the Country Music Hall of Fame.

Their strange mystique derived in part from keeping their lives under wraps. Alvin Pleasant Delaney Carter—a rangy, jug-eared introvert with a mild tremor—had once been married to Sara. The Katharine Hepburn of country music, she wore slacks, went hunting, and smoked cigarettes. A.P. was devoted to her, but his oddball habits and long absences had driven her to divorce him in 1936. She had also fallen in love with A.P.'s cousin, Coy Bays, but the incestuous drama was too much for Coy and he had moved to California, leaving A.P. and Sara still yoked together in the act.

As for Maybelle, Sara's cousin, she mostly kept her head down and played the guitar. A twenty-nine-year-old self-taught virtuoso, Maybelle devised a method of playing melody and rhythm at the same time, anchored by a "bass-string rumble" known as the Carter scratch, which would powerfully influence the next generation of country-music guitarists. "[Sara's] remarkable voice," said a devotee, "A.P.'s vivid song constructions, and Maybelle's treble harmonies and instrumental ability were the act's tickets to immortality."

In Del Rio they joined XERA's four-hour nightly program, "Good Neighbor Get Together." The Carters did an hour, with other slots filled by Cowboy Slim Rinehart, the Prairie Sweethearts, and the Pickard Family from Tennessee. As a family the Pickards were a different species altogether, a raucous, cornpone act partial to tunes like "She'll Be Comin' Round the Mountain" and "Buffalo Gals." And they advertised anything. To the suck and wheeze of an old accordion, Daddy Pickard shilled for Kolorbak and the unsinkable Peruna, which after a couple of recipe revisions down the years now contained eighteen percent alcohol, plus turkey corn, horseweed, cubebs, oil of copaiba, buckthorn, ginger, wild cherry, glycerin, gentian, boneset, potassium iodide, and squills.

The Carter Family did no selling. (They actually preferred another remedy, Hadacol; someone remembered Brinkley fluttering around the edges of the studio, fearful they were going to mention it on the air.) What they did was make music that was unblinking, elemental, sometimes bleak to the bone; it gave comfort by offering no false comfort. It was quite a contrast, Brinkley's calculated maunderings about cowbells at eventide set against the gothic sincerity of the Carters. But it let the world discover what the South already knew. Streaming out under the doctor's glandular banner, their songbook—

"Will the Circle Be Unbroken?" "Wildwood Flower," "Keep on the Sunny Side," and many more—became fixed in America's heart.

On their first trip to Del Rio, Maybelle brought along her youngest daughter, Anita, age five. The little girl was wild with energy; she walked on her hands so much, one family member said, people recognized Anita's butt faster than her face. One day she did a duet on air with her mother, a tune called "Little Buckaroo." This paved the way for more Carter girls to come west: Maybelle's other daughters, Helen and June, and A.P. and Sara's youngest, Janette. All but Janette loved singing on the radio, though the studio rehearsals were a grind. Janette remembered Anita curled up to sleep in a guitar case.

Once Brinkley invited his top act to visit his estate. The Carters were waiting on the mansion's first floor when the doctor appeared unto them accompanied by a friend. "He came down the stairs and he had a monkey on his shoulder with a tail around his neck," Anita said later. "I certainly had never seen anything like that."

Cue female voice husky with longing: "Can men be reacti-vated?"

Cue he-man voice: "Write to the Brinkley Hospitals, Little Rock, Arkansas, and enclose ten cents. . . ."

Arkansas?

They were the perfect couple, or so it seemed, but Brinkley hadn't been home long before he and Del Rio had a falling-out. The fight was over another man: James Middlebrook, a local surgeon who, while Brinkley was summering overseas, began offering knockoffs of his treatments at one-fifth the price. Middlebrook even had the cheek to plug them over a rival border blaster. Brinkley fought back, savaging the thief and impostor on XERA ("Some men have been led astray . . . some have died . . ."). The rivalry grew so spirited that each man hired a gang of thugs to haunt the depot every day and snatch trade as it stepped off the train. Slugfests broke out between the factions. Knives flashed. There were reports of men arriving on other business entirely being bundled into cars and, to the sound of smothered cries, borne off to one doctor or the other. The townspeople took sides. When a Brinkley backer spotted a Middlebrook recruiter outside the Roswell Hotel, he didn't pass by on the other side. "He was trying to rob Dr. Brinkley of his patients," said Henry "Coonie" Crawford, "and I just floored him. He slid halfway up under the car."

Brinkley took the position that after all he had done for Del Rio, the city fathers should drive the poacher out. When they declined to intervene, he yanked his practice and moved it to Little Rock, Arkansas. As often happens with decisions made in anger, he only made life harder for himself. Now he had to commute each week between his hospital in Arkansas and his Mexican radio station. Minnie, who told him all along he was making a mistake, stayed put in their mansion.

The clinic in downtown Little Rock opened on January 28, 1938. Located at the corner of Twentieth Street and Schiller Avenue, it was a sleek glass-and-chrome facility with forty beds and a pharmacy inside. The doctor also took over a bankrupt country club fifteen miles outside of town. Now he could offer convalescents greenery and golf. There was Continental cuisine in the restaurant and a small orchestra in the ballroom where the ambulatory were invited to tango.

Even so, business in Little Rock was merely satisfactory. Brinkley soon realized he could never be a big fish in the big city the way he had been in a backwater. Lately, too, he felt, shooing the flies off Hitler was taking time away from drumming up trade.

A few months after the doctor shifted his health center to Arkansas, Norman Baker did the same. In the town of Eureka Springs (modestly famous for its sixty pools of healing "wonder water"), he took over the Crescent Hotel, a Victorian pile of turrets and gingerbread atop a high hill. He renamed it the Baker Cancer Cure Hospital, painted his office bright purple, hung two submachine guns on the wall, and installed bulletproof windows. The old-lady lobby was recast in red, yellow, orange, and black. Baker even invited the enterprising Dr. Middlebrook, the man who had driven Brinkley out of Del Rio, to come join the new venture in Eureka Springs—a hundred thousand dollars a year, he promised, private plane included. What a thumb in the eye that would have been to the quack who stalked his dreams. But Middlebrook declined.

More and more, Baker's radio talks were shading into right-wing rants.

45

The Little Rock hospital had just opened its doors when, in January and February 1938, Fishbein's two-part "Modern Medical Charlatans" appeared on newsstands. The "filth and falsehood" of Brinkley's career was writ larger than ever before. Now he was "a blatant quack . . . whose professional record reeks with charlatanism of the crudest type," one in whom "quackery reaches its apotheosis. Without anything resembling a real medical education, with licenses purchased and secured through extraordinary manipulations of political appointees, and with consummate gall beyond anything ever revealed by any other charlatan, Brinkley . . . continues to demonstrate his astuteness in shaking shekels from the pockets of credulous Americans."

Every line had the same purpose. Like Holmes pursuing Moriarty, Fishbein was trying to force a showdown, to make Brinkley turn and fight. Reichenbach Falls in this case would be civil court: with U.S. criminal law so woefully weak on killer quacks it was the only possible venue. But to get there Brinkley would have to sue for libel and this time follow through. If he did, if he took the bait, federal court would make that old Kansas medical-board hearing look like a pat on the head and a candy apple.

There was little doubt that the man who had already called the AMA "the biggest bunch of grafters and the biggest bunch of crooks and the biggest bunch of thieves on the top side of this earth" would not appreciate this new smackdown, and indeed for weeks he fumed and complained about it on the radio. But that was all he did, and

Fishbein's gambit seemed to have failed. Two months passed before Brinkley announced he was suing for libel and $250,000 in damages. Viewing the rashness of this choice long afterward, a psychologist wrote: "His protracted struggle with his great nemesis, Morris Fishbein and the American Medical Association, appears in hindsight to have been inevitable, as though he sought persecution deliberately." But then why shouldn't he? For years persecution had been less a source of misery to Brinkley than a wellspring of his power. In 1938 he was one of the best-known doctors in the world, as well as a freshly minted political pundit. Both had reputations to protect. On top of that, he was being increasingly harassed by uppity lawsuits against him by former patients; if he beat his worst critic, slew him in the Coliseum, it would send a message to all those malcontents out there. Third, the trial would be a showdown between an Aryan and a Jew. In Brinkley's cosmology, the outcome could not be in doubt.

Setting all that aside—emotional spurs, strategic incentives, the burning memory of Fishbein on that ship—Brinkley still had good reason to believe he could win. Fishbein's grip on power at the AMA was showing signs of slipping. Insurrectionists in the organization were causing trouble, accusing him of treating *JAMA* as his personal platform and suppressing dissent and debate—his response to which, that he couldn't be expected to make room "for the notions of every nit wit that comes along," had done nothing to help his popularity. A new profile in *Fortune* articulated other cracks in his support: "A good many doctors feel that Dr. Fishbein's [speeches and jokes] are not quite in keeping with the dignity of the profession. . . . Since one of the main ethical tenets of the Association is the prohibition of self-advertising some doctors believe that he puts himself in an ambiguous position by inspiring murder-sized headlines wherever he goes." This wasn't all to the bad; while promoting himself, Fishbein had "promoted the A.M.A. from a mild academic body into a powerful trade association." Still, invaluable though he was, he had "failed to develop in social consciousness as fast as the needs of the day require"—in other words, he hadn't adapted to the crisis of the

Depression. In November 1937, an organization calling itself the Group Health Association (GHA), a cell of AMA members, had formed a medical cooperative in Washington, D.C. ("The idea . . . was to give patients financial relief with prepaid health insurance 'premiums' and to improve the incomes of physicians by paying them fixed salaries from these premiums.") It was managed care in embryo, and the leadership of the AMA, Fishbein included, had responded with flamethrowers, denouncing the plan as "socialized medicine" and threatening its proponents with excommunication if they persisted. Siding with the rebels, the U.S. Department of Justice had indicted Fishbein and twenty others under the Sherman Antitrust Act for restraint of trade.

H. L. Mencken leapt to his friend's defense. In a column he called the insurgents "scurvy liars," adding: "I happen to be well acquainted with Dr. Fishbein. . . . It is my belief that no abler, more honest, more intelligent or more courageous editor is in practice in the United States." In a similar vein, Mencken wrote Assistant U.S. Attorney General Thurman Arnold in August 1938, urging him to call off the case against the AMA: "The onslaught on Fishbein is especially vicious. . . . No man in this country has ever done more to raise the standards of American hospitals, or to protect the American people against patent medicine and other quacks. In the latter field his work has been a hundred times as effective as that of all the reformers on Capitol Hill. It seems to me an outrage that so useful and honest a man should be subjected to such disingenuous attacks, and that the government of the United States should give them countenance."

Small wonder Brinkley saw blood in the water. The more Fishbein was tarred as obstructionist and reactionary, the easier it should be for an alternative healer to crush him in court. It was a delicious moment: for the first time in their long war, Brinkley wasn't the one in trouble with the law.

46

Patsy Montana, the "Cowboy's Sweetheart," didn't like being caught in the middle. But A.P. and Sara Carter had hit another bad patch: they were getting through their shows at night but otherwise not speaking. "Whenever A.P. wanted to say something to Sara," Patsy said, "he'd call me over, and I'd have to relay his message. It sure was awkward."

In February of 1939 something in Sara gave way. These last few months at XERA she had come to realize how big a stage she commanded. One night without warning in the middle of a set, she dedicated the next song to her lost love, Coy Bays, who she hoped was listening in California.

> *It would've been better for us both had we never*
> *In this wide wicked world ever met.*
> *For the pleasures we've both seen together*
> *I am sure, love, we'll never forget.*
> *Oh, I'm thinking tonight of my blue eyes*
> *Who is sailing far over the seas.*
> *Oh, I'm thinking tonight of him only*
> *And I wonder if he ever thinks of me.*

It could not have soothed A.P.'s feelings any that "I'm Thinking Tonight of My Blue Eyes" was a song he had written, or at least massaged together from ancient sources. Coy did hear the broadcast, headed straight for Texas, and he and Sara were married.

Suddenly the Carter Family sounded different on the air. Told nothing, listeners were left to guess the truth: A.P. had walked off. Ordinarily Brinkley would have leapt into a crisis of this magnitude. But now he was otherwise engaged.

February 19, 1939

[To] Morriss and Morriss, Lawyers
National Bank of Commerce Building
San Antonio, Texas

Gentlemen:
Phil Foster [another attorney] is in my office at this writing, and we are discussing the Fishbein article, and I make the following suggestions as to preparation of evidence, witnesses to be had, depositions to be taken, etc.

First, I am not going on the witness stand. I spent fourteen hours on a witness stand in Topeka [at the medical board hearing in 1930], and I know what I'm up against. I do not feel physically able to undergo two or three days of cross examination about immaterial things in this case.

Second, we must open our case and deny each and every one of the allegations made by Fishbein. This will be done by other witnesses than myself, and if they are the right caliber of witnesses they will be more effective before a Judge and jury than the plaintiff, speaking in his own behalf and interested in the case. . . .

We can prove, if you deem necessary, by bringing cured and satisfied patients to the witness stand, that these men had been treated by so-called ethical members of the Medical Association, and had been diagnosed as having a prostate that must be removed, cut out, and that months ago, or years ago they came to me [instead] and have been well ever since. . . .

Much of what Brinkley is saying here makes sense. He quite reasonably wants the jury to hear about the impressive-sounding tests run on customers when they first arrive: "The patient's nose is looked into with electrically lighted instruments, his tonsils are examined, his teeth are trans-illuminated, his rectum is examined [with a] proctoscope and a sigmoidscope, his stomach is examined with barium meals and the X-ray, dyes are given for examination of the gallbladder and the kidneys."

What the letter chiefly reveals, though, is a man in the gravitational pull of Mars. He apparently doesn't realize that as he is the plaintiff in a libel trial, the other side can force him to testify—but that's a detail. Brinkley is so used to treating the truth as raw material that even when preparing for the fight of his life, and under the cloak of attorney-client privilege, he can't stop doing it:

"So far as the indictment in California was concerned, this thing was so simple and ridiculous that the charges were automatically dropped when the investigation got under way. . . .

"In 1925 I went to The Royal University of Pavia, attended the final course in the graduating class and received my diploma. After that I passed the equivalent of a State Board examination in Italy [a test lasting thirteen days, he claimed], and am licensed to practice medicine in Italy, today."

To send his own lawyers into court armed with wishful thinking couldn't be expected to help him, any more than his response to Fishbein's persistent demand that he be prosecuted for mail fraud: "[This] seems to me a serious allegation for Brother Fishbein to prove, because Uncle Sam has thoroughly investigated my mail activities, and found me clean as a hound's tooth." He seems inexplicably confident that the ingredients of potions like his Formula 1020 (blue water) can be shielded as trade secrets: "I believe that my Doctors and Druggist should say that these prescriptions and formulas are the private property of Doctor B, and that they have no authority from Doctor B to divulge their contents."

A lifetime of deceiving others has ended in deceiving himself: "Fishbein was so afraid of me and my wife on shipboard that every time we got near him, he ran away. The man lived in mortal fear of meeting me face to face. One day he was sitting on deck reading a book. I stopped in front of him and gazed at him, and the man actually turned green. A Jew doesn't turn white—he turns green when he is afraid."

47

A half inch of rainfall, the first in many days, had laid the dust and cheered the populace. Now in the gray dawn of March 22, 1939, vendors were setting up their stalls in downtown Del Rio near the corner of Garner and Main. Come noon, the old señora would be doing a brisk business in grease-blotched goat-tripe tacos (three cents each) and heavy glass bottles of Coca-Cola. Somebody else was unpacking straw sombreros and gold-painted belt buckles to tempt the out-of-towners. For yonder in the county courthouse—a three-story stucco building with a red-pipe roof and a fat magnolia tree out front—the curtain was about to rise on *John R. Brinkley* v. *Morris Fishbein,* a show that promised to be the best entertainment seen in these parts since the days when Judge Roy Bean was swinging his gavel at the Jersey Lilly Saloon.

There was more at stake this time than the fate of some horse thief. Today's face-off marked the long-awaited showdown between free-range quackery and medicine's professional mainstream. Or as the *San Angelo Standard Times* succinctly put it, "this trial is to determine whether the American Medical Association shall be the guiding factor in the nation's medical circles, or whether Dr. Brinkley is to skyrocket to even greater than million-dollar-a-year success." A great gulf yawned between the opposing parties—though a stranger might have needed some guidance at first distinguishing the two.

When *Time* magazine referred to "the nation's most ubiquitous, most widely maligned, and perhaps most influential medico," it accurately thumbnailed Brinkley. But it was actually describing Morris

Fishbein in the toils of the antitrust suit against the AMA. Just one more step in the process military strategists call "replication"—the principle whereby great opponents over time grow more and more alike—for by now Brinkley and Fishbein had more in common than either would ever have admitted, especially to themselves. Both had egos the size of a weather balloon. Both were workaholic masters of self-promotion, both brilliant and indefatigable talkers who could hypnotize large groups. Both, it was said, had photographic memories. Both railed against Roosevelt. And each other.

All this common ground fed the common view that the verdict could go either way. Many respectable people agreed with Brinkley that the AMA was monopolistic and intolerant. "What next?" asked a Texas scribe. "*Quién sabe,* in the language of this border city, but nearly all agree that a victory over the American Medical Association would turn loose the greatest publicity barrage the country has ever known for some goal Dr. Brinkley quickly could set. Likewise, [a] Brinkley victory could mean a great setback to the nationwide organization of physicians. . . ." Some observers said a win might put the goat-gland man in the White House.

On the other hand, the *New York Times* now referred to him as "Dr." Brinkley.

About 8:30 A.M. the plaintiff rolled down Main Street toward the courthouse in a long Cadillac driven by his wife. Of all his cars this was his favorite, fire-engine red with DR. BRINKLEY embossed on it in thirteen places. Right behind him came Rose Dawn at the wheel of her pink Chrysler. Brinkley had been asking her recently about his chances of becoming president. The stars were auspicious, she said.

In the dining room of the Roswell Hotel, former site of Brinkley's hospital, Morris Fishbein was still finishing his breakfast. It had been a busy month. In the past few days he had lunched with Somerset Maugham, then triumphed in a Missouri court over 8'11" Robert Wadlow and his family. The parents had sued *JAMA* for portraying the tallest man in the world as mentally and emotionally backward.

Now as he chiseled into his grapefruit, Fishbein scanned some of the mail which had been pouring in from supporters of his war on Brinkley.

From Reverend J. W. Hendrix of Drownfield, Texas: "It get old to hear of piles, hemorrhoids, p[r]ostate glands, of men who have lost their sex interests, of assured rejuvenation, of who begat while rejuvenated, of men who are on the way to join the sisterhood unless they rush in to get a goat gland. . . . [T]here are literally thousands of people who are interested on your behalf. They may not be able to reach you, to help you; yet they're anxious to be relieved, to get all this litter off the air."

From F. W. Bushner of Chicago: "My son took me to Rochester to the Mayo Bros and they saved my life, they told me that they get a lot of Brinkley's patients that Brinkley operated on. . . . I have him to blame for having the ruptured bladder, and another thing I cannot do a day's work on that account, he ruined me."

From Mrs. Samuel Garner of Lincoln, Nebraska: "While in the south [my cousin] contracted malarial fever and being on their return trip home and feeling ill and passing [Brinkley's] hospital he said 'Take me in there.' The result was he became a victim of their prostate gland operation and what all, and died. . . . Upon reading the proof of death the physician under whose care he had been in Blue Island declared 'it was a case of *murder*.' He declared that no reputable physician would operate on a man carrying the blood pressure that this man did. In checking their bank account we found a cancelled check given to the Brinkley Hospital for $1000. What reputable hospital in the United States would make a "cleaning" like that besides killing the man."

Up the street, the courthouse was already crowded inside and out. Judge R. J. McMillan, who ran a tight ship, had announced he would allow no standing room, so when the inner doors opened there was a rush and a musical chairs–style fight for fewer than a hundred seats. When the clamor died down and deputy sheriffs had returned the losers to the hall, more than three-quarters of Brinkley's cheering section proved to be women, drawn by drama and the pull of the alpha male.

Some spots were saved for coots and codgers, about a dozen, recruited by the doctor's attorneys to provide the all-important testimonials. ("They were the friskiest bunch of old roosters you ever saw in your life," said Clinton Giddings Brown, Fishbein's lead attorney, "so we knew what to expect.") The rest of the reserved seats were filled by other witnesses for both sides and Miss Nelson's civics class from the local high school. The boys and girls were on a field trip to observe firsthand the workings of American jurisprudence.

Fishbein checked his watch and stuffed the letters into his briefcase as a waitress was clearing his table. She paused with her laden tray and asked him how it felt to be Brinkley's guest.

The editor didn't understand.

"He's still part owner of this hotel," she said. "And that grapefruit you just ate came from his orchard."

Her look said, Next time bring your own grapefruit.

48

During jury selection Brinkley stood at a side table sipping ice water. One by one they took their places: twelve men, mostly ranchers in string ties and tooled-leather boots with goats of their own at home. Whether their knowledge of this animal would be a minus or a plus for the doctor was an open question, but he knew the locals in general were rooting for him. Even after his defection to Little Rock, most of Del Rio had remained abidingly grateful to him for pulling their town through the Great Depression. They had taken out ads saying so.

Did it bother Fishbein, trying the case in alien territory? From his spot by the water pitcher, Brinkley studied his opposite number, who sat jotting in a small notebook with a gold pen, surrounded by five lawyers. *Five*. That didn't look like confidence. To Brinkley—and to others in the room—it looked like arrogance, overspending, and probably fear. In fact Fishbein's lead attorney, Clinton Giddings Brown, was privately worried about it himself: that next to Brinkley's homegrown father-and-son legal team, this muscle flexing by "jealous doctordom" would work against his client—just as back in 1930 that hostile combine of the AMA, the medical board, and the *Kansas City Star* had almost put Brinkley in the governor's mansion. Well, Brown thought, it was done now. At least he himself would be handling most of the witnesses, something he was adept at, and he knew how to rub a jury's belly now and then. A former mayor of San Antonio and now a powerhouse in Houston, Brown had written a book for boys about

235

the Alamo, and he took care to come across as a gallus-popper of the old school.

"All rise."

Over the course of the next week—leaving aside the testimony of the principals—the two sides seemed evenly matched. At least that's how the crowd in the courtroom saw it, but then most of them backed the doc. Effie Kelly took the stand first. Owner of a Del Rio newsstand, she was called by the plaintiff's lawyers to prove that the offending magazine had reached the public. Other witnesses followed to say they had read Fishbein's extraordinary charges—a man in the ice business, for example, who had stayed at the Gunter Hotel in San Antonio, "and that is where I seen this article, this magazine, and read it; it was laying on the dresser in the hotel room just about in the position I have it in my hand, right now."

After that, some of Brinkley's medical staff took the stand to vouch for his work. This task fell chiefly to Dr. A. C. Petermeyer, a self-anointed osteopath who was part of Brinkley's inner circle. Richly attired, Petermeyer had a round face, an aspirant mustache, and eyes that burned like a holy man's, perhaps because he was scared of his boss's lawyer. An old junkyard dog skilled at savage cross-examination, Will Morriss Sr. sometimes seemed resentful when he had to ask friendly questions, as if he might suddenly throw off all restraint and tear apart his own witness.

Petermeyer confirmed that Dr. Fishbein's article had humiliated Dr. Brinkley and kept him indoors more than usual. But Morriss wanted something else, too. To counter portrayals of his client as a humbug, which he knew of course were coming, he wanted to pre-emptively paint Brinkley as the most exacting of scientists, the most careful of surgeons, the most learned of men, and how better (as Brinkley himself had long shown) than to cloud men's minds with jargon? Petermeyer loyally supplied it: "The scrotum is anesthetized with apothsine. . . . The testicle is picked up in the left hand with the index finger of the right hand; the head of the epididymis is an appendage of the testicle; and an incision is made through the skin, through the dartos, through the fascia, through the cremasteric muscle. . . .

"My experience with at least a thousand [prostate] cases," he added, "has been that ninety per cent of the patients treated and operated on by the ligature method were improved, some were completely relieved of their symptoms and some only partially, and those that received partial relief were those of advanced enlargements where the transurethral resection was also used to bring about the desired result."

While Minnie paced and fretted in the hall, occasionally peeking her head in the door, Brinkley sat at the counsel table watching the proceedings like Patience on a monument. Clustered behind him was his personal support team from the radio station: Rose Dawn, singer Rosa Dominguez ("the Mexican Nightingale"), and others. Observing him, Fishbein later described Brinkley as "a little man with a little goatee, wearing a gray suit. . . . He sat quietly in the courtroom, usually chewing a toothpick and combing his beard with his fingers. In his vest pocket he carried a combination gold tooth and ear pick, with which he used to explore his teeth, his nose, his ears, and then view the results with a tender expression."

Before leaving the stand, Petermeyer was asked to explain why his boss sent prostate patients home with extra ampules of Formula 1020—the first mention of what would become a bitter issue at the trial. The witness explained that this medicine was a personal creation of Dr. Brinkley's, designed to fight infection by boosting the patient's white-blood-cell count.

After that, five more of Brinkley's employees testified fulsomely to his skill. Dr. J. H. Davis, on staff since 1933, said, "I wouldn't know the exact percentage, but the percent [of prostate patients] relieved is very large," based on dozens of follow-ups he himself had conducted. Dr. Leslie Dye Conn claimed that 90 percent showed improvement. As the trial progressed, and experts for both sides trooped to the stand, a growing gallery of explanatory diagrams (including cross sections of the penis and prostate) appeared on blackboards and a wall by the witness box. It soon became clear that for the boys and girls of

Miss Nelson's class, the workings of justice had been eclipsed as a subject of interest.

Cross-examining members of Brinkley's medical staff, Clinton Brown made some headway impeaching their credentials, integrity, or both. But one of them undermined his employer more subtly, and unintentionally, by providing a frank picture of the level of talent Brinkley attracted. Neither a crook nor a true believer, Otis Chandler (no relation to the *Los Angeles Times* editor) presented himself just as he was, a very average man fighting to survive the Depression:

> I was left stranded down at San Antonio with a wife and three kids, and I started in trying to make a living in South Texas, and there was next to nothing to start with, and I bucked the game over at the little town of Weslaco in the Winter Garden the best I could, and then I went to Karnes City, and from there to Poteet and finally into San Antonio, and in my messing around when I stopped at Karnes City for a spell I met a young fellow by the name of Alvis working in a drug store there, and I got him out of a rut and got him started, and he happened to drive into Del Rio and start working for Jim Shearn over here in a drug store, and Dr. Brinkley's x-ray man flew the coop for some unknown reason, I don't know why, and this boy knew my financial straits and he wanted me to come over and do x-ray work because he heard that I did that, and that is how I got there.

When court adjourned that first day, Brinkley made straight for his studio over the J. C. Penney store, pulled his chair up to the microphone, and started talking. He had just thought of a new contest, he said, top prize five hundred dollars, to the listener who best completed this phrase in twenty words or less: "I consider Dr. Brinkley the world's foremost prostate specialist because . . ."

Then, after some airy remarks about the trial, he ended with: "If Dr. Fishbein goes to heaven, I want to go the other way."

Next morning infuriated defense attorneys tried to have him cited for contempt, accusing Brinkley of making mock of the proceedings and trying to influence members of the jury (who were not sequestered) after hours. But the judge didn't view it that seriously, and Brinkley went on running radio contests each night of the weeklong trial.

That was a minor dustup compared with what happened next, when Will Morriss turned to Brinkley's roster of coots—the old men lined up to testify in all their rejuvenated glory.

First up was rancher I. F. "Frenchy" Ingram, lively as a grig, ready to recount how Dr. Brinkley had cured his crippling rheumatism. Approaching the witness stand, Ingram spun on his right foot and slid smoothly into the chair. He identified himself as a former patient of the plaintiff's. That was as far as he got.

Clinton Brown said, "I object."

The wrangling that followed was loud and long, the most rancorous of the trial. Insisting, with slaps on the table, that the accounts of these former patients were "a matter of the utmost importance" to his client, Will Morriss cited Brinkley's medical-board hearing in 1930, when patients both satisfied and otherwise had told their stories at length. Morriss apparently believed that the rules followed in Kansas would also apply here. Unfortunately—to quote a young girl in a film of that year—they weren't in Kansas anymore.

Brown argued that federal-court rules were stricter than the ad hoc accommodations of a medical board, which wasn't even a court at all. An example of *legal* precedent, Brown said, would be the long-standing evidentiary rule that prevented nonexperts from offering expert opinion: in this case, laymen passing judgment on medical procedures. Judge McMillan took a long night to think it over. Next morning he announced his decision.

Gentlemen, I am of the opinion that the specific instances of malpractice couldn't be shown, nor could specific instances of good result obtained by [Brinkley] be shown. . . . [If the attempt were made], it would open up an unlimited field of evidence in which, maybe, seventy-five or a hundred patients might appear and, for some reason or other, claim they had been benefited, and seventy-five or a hundred might appear on the other side and claim they had been mistreated or hadn't been benefited, and the first thing you know the trial would deteriorate from a trial of issues before the court and jury to one of prejudice and passion and feeling. . . . I don't think that that kind of evidence is admissible.

At a stroke, Brinkley's twenty witnesses were out. Next recess Clinton Brown stood outdoors watching them depart: "The whole bunch of them went down the steps together, some with heads bowed and all walking as if they were going to a funeral." Of course excluding the coots and codgers meant that the maimed and aggrieved couldn't testify either, but Brown had planned all along to fight on a narrower patch of ground.

Faced with a major setback, Will Morriss tried to twist it to his advantage, making the improbable claim that if Brinkley's testimonials were out, then the opinions of Fishbein's experts should be excluded, too. On the contrary, the judge sardonically replied; those experts were crucial to finding out whether Brinkley's reputation had been harmed, for "if it happens he had no standing in the opinion of his fellow doctors [before Fishbein's article appeared], it follows naturally he hasn't been damaged."

Whereupon three eminent Texas urologists—A. I. Folsom of Dallas; Manning Venable of San Antonio; B. Weems Turner of Houston—denounced Brinkley in turn, flourishing pointers at charts. All the witnesses said Brinkley's prostate treatments were valueless at best and that the goat-gland transplant was nonsense. Legal tacticians noted that Brown kept returning to goats and gonads as the subject most ripe for ridicule, despite strenuous and ongoing objections from Morriss that all this was "irrelevant and immaterial," since the transplants had stopped six years ago. The more McMillan allowed the questioning, the madder plaintiff's attorneys got.

JUDGE: I think you have indicated, counsel, your objection to this line of procedure. [The record is preserved.] If you want to keep bobbing up you have the right to do it.

MORRISS: We said we didn't want to do it.

JUDGE: You said you didn't want to do it, but you keep doing it.

As for Brinkley's vaunted Formula 1020, it was exposed as nothing more than colored water, which one urologist said made it worse than worthless: "Distilled water is considered a bad thing to inject by itself into the blood stream. . . . Because of the fact that it is a weaker solution, it tends to absorb out of the blood cells certain substances which are necessary for their proper functioning, and therefore the distilled water is considered not only not a beneficial but an actively harmful thing."

After Fishbein's trio of experts, James E. Crawford appeared.

Not in the flesh. Brinkley's old electro-medic partner couldn't be present because he was again serving time. What Fishbein's attorneys did introduce, however, was a 1930 deposition in which he detailed his criminal escapades with Brinkley, leading up to their flight from Greenville. Choice portions were read aloud for the delectation of the jury, including Crawford's description of Brinkley injecting "sweetened water" into his patients twenty-six years earlier—back in what the doc liked to call "the valley of yesterday." They had "innumerable applications for treatment," Crawford said, which they supplied for about two months and then skipped town.

Q: Was there any particular reason for not paying your bills?

A: We probably would have been wise if we had, but we didn't 'cause we wanted the money.

49

When late in the week Morris Fishbein took the stand in his own defense, he was a hyperactive model of serenity and reason. He had not been in the witness chair more than five minutes before Judge McMillan admonished him for talking too fast, even while he pitched himself (with some success) as a messenger of truth above the fray.

Questioned by Brown, he sketched the august history of the AMA and his own credentials as a quack buster. Then he was asked how he felt about Brinkley.

"My feelings would be, from a scientific point of view, quite negative," Fishbein said blandly, though he harbored no "personal animosity." A vendetta? That was absurd. Rather, one might view his campaign against "Mr. Brinkley" as a sort of surgical procedure, "like dissecting away a malignant tumor from a normal body, and off the body of science." He glanced at the tumor himself seated across the way.

Then Brown took Fishbein through his inflammatory magazine article point by point, identifying sources for his allegations and justifying his choice of words ("the apotheosis of quackery"). Some of his statements, Fishbein said, were based on the "admitted biography" of Brinkley, Clement Wood's notorious *Life of a Man*. Some came from material collected by Arthur Cramp at the Bureau of Investigation, some from published interviews with victimized patients, some from listening to him on the radio. Fishbein explained yet again how Brinkley displayed the classic hallmarks of a quack: the impossible promises, the "trade secrets," the long list of fake degrees. Real doctors share real discoveries because they want to help people, he said, whereas Brinkley's so-called discoveries have "never been published in any medical periodical nor . . . submitted to the criticism of the medical profession," and for good reason. His vaunted Formula 1020 would have stood revealed as nothing more than plain water with "an infinitesimal, a very tiny amount of coloring matter," so small the AMA lab had to bring in a microchemist to figure out what it was.

And what was it?

"Approximately one drop of indigo to 100,000 parts of water— about what you would get by throwing a bottle of bluing into Lake Michigan." Each ampule had cost about eighteen cents to manufacture; Brinkley sent each of his prostate patients home with a half dozen, for which he charged one hundred dollars—a markup of more than 9,200 percent. And this was just one example! The recklessness of *Medical Question Box*, the comedy and tragedy of goat glands, all of Brinkley's vulpine machinations for more than twenty years had been directed toward a single goal: self-aggrandizement, financial, egoistic, any kind you cared to name. He himself, Fishbein said, because of his unique position at the AMA, was personally acquainted with more than ten thousand physicians in America, and he had never known one of them to have a gross income in excess of a million dollars, the amount Brinkley admitted taking in during 1937. "That's not medical practice," the editor concluded. "That's big business."

All right, said Brown, but how could he be so sure that Brinkley's rejuvenation techniques were worthless? Well-respected men, both in Europe and the United States, had been claiming success with similar methods for many years.

With a settled sigh Fishbein faced the jury. Reversing the natural aging process, he said, was no more possible than restoring "the elasticity in a pair of suspenders." Rejuvenation was a snare and a delusion from which the public, he prayed, was at long last beginning to awake.

"Your witness."

. . .

Over the next several hours Will Morriss conducted such a snarling, snapping cross-examination he suggested, however faintly, the need for animal control. Stripped of digressions and repetitions, it went like this:

Q: You had opportunities to discuss with Dr. Brinkley his methods, had you wanted to?

A: Had I wanted to, yes, sir.

Q: You never made any investigation at all?

A: Personally, no.

Q: Never made any effort to contact Dr. Brinkley?

A: Personally, no, sir.

Q: You never made any effort to learn of him about his practice and his operations or his reasons for it, or anything about that?

A: I made no personal effort.

Q: Why did you decline the opportunity time after time?

A: In some twenty-six years of investigations of charlatans, I have never met personally or sought the acquaintance of any charlatan.

Q: Do you mean to sit there on the witness stand and assert that Dr. Brinkley is a charlatan?

A: I do.

Morriss fingered his notes.

Q: Are you in any way committed by any authority, governmental or other authority with the power to say who may practice medicine in the United States and who may not?

A: No, sir.

Q: Do you set yourself up to?

A: No, sir.

Q: When did you first read this book which charged you with attempting to be the "Mussolini of Medicine" in America?

A: I read that about, I think, the first time a month ago maybe.

Q: And shortly before that there was a great controversy and furor in the medical profession about a good many of your methods, wasn't there?

A: No, sir.

Q: Hadn't there been a great deal of dissension about it, so much so that you have had some trouble up at Washington lately that is due to some of your practices?

A: No, sir.

Q: You were recently indicted in the federal court in Washington, and you are under indictment now?

A: Yes, sir.

Q: And that was due to your methods, what many doctors called your high-handed methods in dealing with and trying to control the medical profession?

A: No, sir.

Q: What was the indictment for, against you?

A: The indictment had to do with the fact that certain hospitals in the District of Columbia—

Q: *Answer the question,* what was the charge made?

JUDGE: He was answering the question. I very much doubt the admissibility of this line of evidence, anyhow. . . . From the court's standpoint the evidence is inadmissible; I think it is prejudicial. . . . We can't try the case in Washington.

Q: I realize that but—

JUDGE: I think you had better discontinue this line of testimony.

Q: My thought was only with reference to his activities.

JUDGE: He is not being tried in regard to that. I have no doubt that he has his side of that thing in Washington. Gentlemen of the jury, you will disregard all of that with regard to this indictment, it has nothing to do with this case and is a collateral issue, and you have no business to try it out, you must discard it from your mind, and I mean for the jury to do that. . . . It is not material and you are not interested in it, so you will not discuss that matter in regard to the indictment or refer to it or carry it in your minds.

Though he must have known he might lose the battle over testimonials, this second blow seemed to catch Morriss flat-footed. The weapon he had counted on, perhaps more than any other, to expose the witness as a hidebound, high-handed bully—an enemy of freedom fighters like Brinkley and those plucky doctors in Washington—had been snatched from his hand.

Morriss took more than a moment to collect himself. When he pressed on, he confronted Fishbein with phrases from the article and staccato demands for proof. "You send in a dollar, he sends you a pill." What was the basis for that calumny?

A: I might have had some material of that sort.
Q: Is that the best excuse you can give?
A: I don't conceive of it as an excuse.
Q: I am asking if that is your best excuse for publishing that?
A: I don't conceive of it as an excuse.
Q: I didn't ask you that.
A: Yes you did.

Dr. Fishbein had made a career of insulting the plaintiff's expertise. What about his own? How many years' experience did Dr. Fishbein have as a practicing physician? One year? A single year? He did say one year? And when was that? In 1912 and 1913. In the witness's opinion, had there been any advances in medicine since before the Great War?

Q: Dr. Fishbein, have you ever performed a prostate operation?
A: No.
Q: Have you ever seen Dr. Brinkley perform a prostate operation?

A: No.

Q: Have you ever talked to or interviewed one of Brinkley's patients?

A: No.

Q: So these writings of yours were based on no personal investigation, no contact with Dr. Brinkley, no patients, no staff. Even on the boat, when he stood not five feet away from you, this most dangerous quack on earth as you claim, you made no effort to engage him?

A: Various investigations [of him] have been made.

Q: I didn't ask you that. . . . Aren't you violating the so-called tenets of the AMA, Dr. Fishbein, by advertising your own works?

A: I don't—

Q: What about this book of yours, *Modern Medical Home Remedies*? Is this not exactly the same formula or concept underlying *Medical Question Box*? . . . Wasn't there considerable furor and criticism within the AMA when you published it?

A: There was some excitement, yes, sir.

Morriss ended with a bang. Had not the AMA's scorched-earth policy against quacks destroyed legitimate physicians as well? Had not organized medicine since the dawn of time tormented and mocked its greatest pioneers? And always the refrain:

That is the best you can give us on that, is it?
That is the best excuse you can give as to that statement?

A bit self-satisfied, insufficiently enterprising perhaps: Fishbein departed with spots on his hat. Nevertheless, as scorekeepers noted, the central thesis of his writings—that Brinkley's medical procedures were worthless—stood unrefuted. In any case few had expected the case to rise or fall with Fishbein. How Brinkley performed—how aggrieved and majestic a figure he cut—that would tell the tale.

50

He looked so chipper at first, glancing about the room like a newly perched bird. Nothing hinted that over the next two days he would wind up assisting at an autopsy on his own career.

The questioning by his attorney was predictably smooth. Brinkley painted his childhood and early professional struggles in sepia, something he could do almost automatically, though he toned down the poetry for court:

Q: And what were the circumstances, Doctor? Were you poor?
A: While father lived we had plenty to eat. After my father died, why, it was a case of root pig or die, and there wasn't very much soil to root in. We were poor. . . .

When Morriss brought him to the subject of Fishbein's article, the famous voice trembled. "It made me feel ashamed," he said, "and it made my wife feel ashamed." As a result of the slurs and lies published there, his income had dropped from "eleven hundred thousand dollars" (he skirted the word *million*) in 1937 to $810,000 in 1938.

But what about these terrible deeds of which he stood accused? The assertion of this low criminal, James Crawford, for example, that he gave hypos of colored water to the good people of Greenville?

"I did not administer any colored water to any patients," Brinkley said quietly, as if weary of confronting this preposterous canard. He had gone to North Carolina all those years ago at the behest of "a

Dr. Burke" in Tennessee to open an office for him there, with the understanding Burke himself would be arriving shortly to take it over. When after weeks of waiting—during which he encountered this James Crawford, a man previously unknown to him—Dr. Burke still had not appeared, Brinkley had caught a train out of town "after telegraphing him that I was leaving."

Q: Did this felon Crawford ever resurface?

A: Yes. He came to see me in Milford during the summer of 1932 while I was a candidate for the governor of the state of Kansas.

Q: He was at large then? He had gotten out of prison?

A: He told me he was out.

Q: Did he tell you how he got out?

A: He told me that while he was an inmate in the penitentiary at McAlester, Oklahoma, he was called into the warden's office where he met two attorneys who introduced themselves to him and told him they were from the American Medical Association and that they wanted a certain deposition from him that would be injurious to me and if he would give them the deposition they would assist him in getting out of the penitentiary. And he said that they gave him a box of cigars and candies and $20 and left, and two weeks later they came back and he gave the kind of deposition they wanted.

Q: What did he propose to you?

A: He told me if I would give him three hundred dollars he would make another deposition saying the one he gave them was all a lie.

Q: What did you tell him?

A: I told him to get the hell out of my office.

All week Morriss had battled every mention of goat glands, and all week he had failed. By now he apparently thought his client would be better off talking about the subject himself, on his own terms, and for his part the doctor seemed delighted to do it. He never tired of reciting the "amazing and startling" results he had achieved, going all the way back to Bill Stittsworth, "who incidentally furnished his own goat."

Q: And then?

A: Of course the news got around in a great fashion, and a cousin of Stittsworth came to me and asked me to do the same thing on him and I did and he had me do transplant glands into his wife. Then one of their relatives was in the insane hospital in Nebraska. He was a banker up there, he was a cashier and lost his mind and had been placed in an insane institution. They wanted to know from me if I thought glands would do this insane person any good, and I said, "Lord God, no," and they said, "We want you to try it" because he had been a masturbator . . . and they brought him down there, took him out of the institution, and I put those glands into him and that man recovered his mind and today is in charge of one of the biggest banks in Kansas City, Missouri. . . . I published that in an article in a little magazine, and down in Alabama a lady read it. She had a daughter that had been in the insane asylum for ten years in Tuscaloosa, Alabama. She was violently insane at times. They had to keep her in what is called a padded cell to keep her from doing injury to herself; she was trying all the time to commit suicide. And my wife and I met this lady with her daughter and brought her over to Milford. I transplanted glands into that young lady. She stayed in my hospital for a month, fully recovered her mental capacity. She secured a secretarial position in Kansas City, Missouri, and married a physician and today she is healthy and happy and normal. I can go on and recite instances like that one after the other. . . .

Q: Now did you or not from your experimentation, your operations, your efforts, your research, did you become convinced that there was benefit in glandular transplantation?

A: I did, I thought I had made a wonderful discovery, I thought this was the grandest thing in the world. I wanted the whole world to know about it.

Only when the AMA refused to publish his findings, he said, did he turn to advertising them himself. He knew of course this would further inflame his enemies, but his duty was clear; the breakthrough he had made was simply "too good and too valuable to keep quiet." As it happened, the pamphlets and handbills were almost superfluous. Once word got out, goat glands sold themselves. "I never tried to produce any patients over the radio at all," he said, "never even made any effort to."

If the technique was so wonderful, why had he abandoned it?

An injectable emulsion had replaced it which worked just as well. Besides, he had hardly given up on goat glands. Once he discovered that they helped men with enlarged prostates urinate more easily—"that was the thing that caught my attention first"—his researches had swept him in that direction, toward ways of treating prostate problems without surgery. Despite the AMA's reckless enthusiasm for it, "removing the prostate gland either superpubically or transurethrally carries with it a certain amount of surgical risk, a danger of hemorrhage, shock, infection. So I started taking out a part of the arteries, the vas deferens artery, tying it off. . . ." It was difficult to explain the process in ways a layman could understand. "This takes the brake off of the substance called prolan in the anterior part of the pituitary gland. . . ."

Q: Doctor, you have heard what was testified by the experts with reference to the physiological impossibility of your prostate treatment benefiting people. What have you got to say about that?

A: I know it does benefit people. When a man has been practicing something for more than twenty years like I have, like I have with thousands of patients, examining those patients when they come to see me the first time and seeing them down through the years . . . why, there isn't any question about the people being helped. . . . My ambition has always been to do all the good that I can in all the ways that I can, and I felt like if I could have introduced something to the medical profession, or the world in general, that would save men from a dangerous surgical operation or loss of their glands that it was worth any sacrifice or anything that I could do to accomplish it, and I still feel the same way today.

"Take the witness," Morriss said, and Clinton Brown stood up. But before he took a step, Judge McMillan interrupted with a warning—not to Brown but to Brinkley—that would frame the contest to come: "A man that comes into a libel trial practically puts his entire life at issue."

The doctor looked unfazed. As a healer he had compelled the gratitude of thousands. He had stood on political platforms and felt worship coming at him in waves. Could anyone so lionized, so canonized, believe himself entirely a quack?

51

Q: Doctor, you have been the possessor of three fine yachts, haven't you?

A: Well, I am happy—

Q: I say, you have been the possessor of three fine yachts, haven't you?

A: I own three yachts, yes, sir.

Q: Well, how many men does it take to run the one you have now?

A: It takes twenty-one men.

Q: A seagoing yacht?

A: Yes, sir.

Q: You don't want to say it is a fine yacht, do you?

A: The one I have now is a mighty nice yacht, yes, sir.

Q: Thank you. Now, when you go and come across the seas on your summer trips you go in the finest boats, don't you?

A: I try to go on good boats, seaworthy boats.

Q: Are there any better boats than the *Queen Mary* or the *Normandie*?

A: If there were, I would have been on them.

Q: You go on the finest boats and stop in the best suite on the boats, don't you?

A: I try to, yes, sir.

Back at the defense table, Brown picked up a copy of Fishbein's article, located a phrase, and read aloud: "'He continues to demonstrate his astuteness in shaking shekels from the pockets of credulous Americans, notwithstanding the efforts of the various governmental departments and agencies.'"

Brinkley waited.

Q: Now as to this article in the *Hygeia,* published by the American Medical Association, it is a fact, is it not, Doctor, that the newspapers and magazines of this country on several occasions have commented most unfavorably about you and your work?

A: I think that what adverse criticism that I have read in the magazines and newspapers concerning me has probably had its basis in statements from the American Medical Association, which they used as an authority in denouncing me.

Q: Do you think most of the men of the American Medical Association instead of being Christian gentlemen as of old, they are politicians and abortionists, do you think that is what the members of the American Medical Association do?

MORRISS: Objection.

JUDGE: Sustained.

It was one of the few successful objections Morriss lodged over the next two long days. But he never stopped trying. While Brown set about disassembling the witness in a lazy, faux-meandering style—idly curious, as it were, about his outbursts of violence, his shady degrees, his lost licenses, the depredations of *Medical Question Box*—Morriss bounced up and down objecting to almost everything, sowing all the confusion he could. Neither attorney threw Brinkley off stride. Whatever his original fears had been about taking the stand, they seemed to have disappeared; he looked serenely prepared, even happy, to handle anything Fishbein's attorney might throw at him.

No cross, no crown.

Q: Complete in twenty words or less: "I consider good health my most valuable possession because . . ." "I consider Dr. Brinkley the world's foremost prostate surgeon because . . ." This is you speaking, sir, two or three nights past on the radio. "All you have to do is think a little and be real sincere and real honest and complete that on one sheet. On the second sheet I want you to mail at least five names and addresses of men that you are personally acquainted with. Be sure you know them, be sure you know they are sick, and be sure you know that they are in need of Brinkley's hospital service. Be sure you know that they are physically and financially able to come to see us. . . . First prize $100, second $50, third $25, fourth $10, five prizes of $5 each, and then 290 other cash awards of $1 each; 299 cash awards." Is it usual for practitioners of medicine in the United States to conduct these prize contests?

A: No, sir, I don't think so.

Q: Do you know of anybody else sending out certificates with red seals on them, telling them, if you will come down to the hospital and write the best piece of any ten people we will put a seal on it like a notary seal and give you an Oldsmobile?

A: No, I don't know of anybody doing that.

Q: Isn't it a fact that the papers all over the country carried pieces about your alleged fakery, quackery and fraudulent activities?

A: I suppose many papers did.

MORRISS: Objection.

JUDGE: Overruled.

Q: Isn't it a fact that you became branded from end to end of the land as a diploma mill graduate?

MORRISS: Objection.

JUDGE: Overruled.

Q: Isn't it a fact that Henry Ford's *Dearborn Independent* called you the dean of quacks?

MORRISS: We object to that as being immaterial and irrelevant and improper and incompetent.

JUDGE: Counsel, I ruled on your matter. You and I have an entirely different conception of the ruling with regard to preserving your record. I think if you make it clearly known to the court that you object to a certain line of procedure and the court overrules you and announces that that line of procedure is to go on, you have done enough. You seem to think you have to get up and make an objection every time a question is asked. . . .

MORRISS: I think this was a different question.

JUDGE: The point about it is, it is militating against the trial in two ways. In the first place, it is taking a lot of time and, in the second place, it is so breaking up the thread of what ought to be brought out that the jury and court and everybody else loses the natural continuity of the story. . . . I have gone to the trouble several times to outline to you my idea as to what I think the course of the trial ought to be. . . . I ruled they could inquire into the money he made out of these operations that were a part of his advertising campaign. . . .

MORRISS: We were under the wrong impression a while ago.

JUDGE: I know, but there doesn't seem to be any way to get rid of you. Every time I say something it provokes a new argument out of you.

MORRISS: Well, I didn't want to be put in the attitude of waiving any matters, and secondly, with reference to this, we thought it was an entirely different matter. . . .

JUDGE: That is the fifth time you told me it was a new matter. If you think that is helping us to go forward, I don't see it.

MORRISS: We except to the court's remark. . . .

The labyrinth of Brinkley's self-justifications Brown rarely approached. Instead he relied on ridicule and hard science. As he had with past witnesses, he repeatedly returned to the subject of goat glands, exploring it in tones of mock respect, like a man hopelessly but sincerely trying to understand the theory of relativity.

Q: Were you the first man that ever did this operation of taking the goat testicle and putting it in the man's testicle?

A: So far as I know I was, yes, sir.

MORRISS: Now of course we just have to object—

JUDGE: Well, if you think it improves your situation any, do it. . . .
It isn't helping the trial along any. . . .

Q: As I understand it, and please correct me if I haven't got it right,
you didn't remove any of the testicles out of the man, did you?

A: The ordinary goat gland operation is what you are thinking
about, isn't it?

Q: Yes.

A: Certain ones I took and cut a hole out of the man's testicle and
took a chunk out and filled the hole up in the testicle with the
goat gland.

Q: Ordinarily you would cut a little flap or slip?

A: Just a pocket to put the gland in.

Q: Would you put a piece of the goat gland in that little hole?

A: No. A three-week-old goat, I would use a three-week-old
gland, just take the capsule off of the gland and transplant the
whole gland.

Q: You would put a goat testicle in one man's testicle and another
on the other side?

A: Yes, and sometimes put them in the abdominal muscles. There
were different locations for them.

[*A stir of surprise in the room.*]

Q: You say now that this was experimental or do you say that it
was the greatest remedy you ever found?

A: I believe that the transplantation of glands is one of the greatest adjuncts to treatment for certain things we have, and I find
that those glands are far superior even today than any product
I can get. . . .

Brown jumped to Formula 1020. Colored water in 1913, colored
water today . . . Might one call it a running constant in his career?

Brinkley, with a burst of spirit this time, denied giving colored
water to anyone.

Brown held up a lab report.

When did things change? When did the moment come when even his greatest supporters could no longer sustain the illusion that he would prevail? By the start of the second day of cross-examination, it was clear that barring a miracle the winner here was foreordained— much like one of those bullfights just over the river, except that in this *plaza de toros* the bull had to sit there while the swords accumulated in his neck.

Brown passed the report to Don Reynolds, another of Fishbein's attorneys, who took over the questioning on Formula 1020. Brinkley repeated Petermeyer's assertion that the medicine was "defensive in its action," that it fought off infection by increasing the number of white blood cells.

Q: I want to know how 1020 produces the white blood cells.

A: It evidently stimulates the thing that makes them.

Q: It does?

A: That is what it causes, and we don't know what causes it, but something . . .

Q: That's your entire explanation?

A: We inject in the patients various vaccines and serums to stimulate the human forces and body against the diseases. . . . I don't think anybody knows what happens or takes place.

Q: What percentage of hydrochloric acid is in the stomach?

A: I will declare, I don't remember. One point two five, I believe, but I forget.

Reynolds challenged the witness to name anyone else, a single physician outside his own staff, who had adopted his "revolutionary" prostate treatments. As Brinkley groped for an answer, Reynolds impatiently pushed on: "Tell me, do you measure the dosage of Formula 1020 by weight or by volume?"

The question caught Brinkley short. He looked here, there, and then out the window as if searching for the answer in the street. It was the longest silence of the trial. Finally he answered. "I wouldn't rightly know that. I don't try to know all the details of what is in this stuff. . . ."

The moment resonated like a gong. Then Clinton Brown rose with a copy of Brinkley's authorized biography, *Life of a Man*. "Interesting reading," Brown began, "if you've got a strong stomach. . . ."

He leafed through the volume shaking his head. Where to begin . . . ?

"'In his mental make-up, he falls exactly into the genius type.'

"'You will . . . find in Dr. Brinkley this lovable characteristic of genius, that money is not an aim, or an end in itself, but a means of enlarging the central idea of his life-work.'

"'God's voice speaking within him . . . The spirit he has can point the way to our salvation. . . . A magnificent radio personality . . . he modulates his voice exquisitely. . . . J. R. BRINKLEY REFUSES PRESIDENCY OF U.S. . . .'"

Q: Doctor, quite truthfully, in your own estimation, are you the greatest prostatic specialist in the world?

A: You know, I certainly don't think so. I imagine there are many men who are probably greater than I am.

Q: Are you the most learned physician in the United States?

A: No sir, I don't think so.

Q: Well, this chapter in your book here, isn't it a fact Chapter Nine is entitled "The Most Learned Doctor in America"?

A: It may be. It may be what Mr. Wood put in it, that biography.

Q: "Dimly he had begun to realize that he was gifted beyond the run of doctors. . . ." Isn't that in your book?

A: Maybe. I don't remember.

Q: And here on page 200, doesn't it say, "I'm going to show the American Medical Association, and the doctors and people of this country, that John R. Brinkley has more medical knowledge than any of them have shown"?

A: I never said it. Probably Wood did.

Q: "In his presentation of facts, no matter on what subject, he is a student of human nature, a psychologist, a master showman, as well as one of the world's most learned doctors and surgeons." Isn't that in your book?

MORRISS: We object to counsel continuously putting into the question "your book."

Q: Where did the man get the facts from that wrote this book?

A: Well, he collected them up from different places. I employed him to write a biography of myself. I paid him to write it. . . .

Q: "The United States government has a legal record for persecution that stinks to Heaven." Has the American government itself been against you?

A: Well, I wouldn't know how to answer that question. . . .

Q: You claim that the president interested himself with the radio commission to get your license revoked, isn't that a fact?

A: Yes, sir. That was told to me by Vice President Curtis. . . .

Q: Did the Kansas Court of Appeals write this about you: ". . . an empiric without moral sense—"?

MORRISS: Objection.

JUDGE: Overruled.

Q: ". . . an empiric without moral sense. . . . Having acted according to the ethical standards of an imposter the licensee has performed an organized charlatanism until he is capable of preying on human weakness, ignorance and credulity to an extent quite beyond the invention of the humble mountebank. . . . By virtue of a license obtained by fraud, the imposter holding it is fleecing the defective, the ailing, the gullible and the chronic medicine-takers, who are moved by suggestion and is scandalizing the medical profession and exposing it to contempt and ridicule." Was this the opinion of the Kansas Court of Appeals regarding you and your work?

A: Something like that. . . .

Q: Doctor, may I ask what is the value of that enormous ring on your left hand there?

A: I paid $4,300 for that ring, sir.

Q: How about the one on your right hand?

A: That ring is worth about $1,000.

Q: How about your stickpin?

A: Fifteen hundred dollars.

Q: Your tie clasp?

A: Oh, about $800.

Q: How many automobiles is it you have now, Doctor?

A: I will have to go to counting up.

MORRISS: I don't know that that has anything to do with the question of this libel suit. . . . If the gentleman thinks he can get some prejudice in that way I don't want to make any particular objection.

JUDGE: Well, if you don't want to object you ought not to rise to your feet. If you want to object the court will rule on it.

Q: How many times does your name appear on your red Cadillac outside?

A: I don't know.

The final thrust was this exchange, when Brown returned to the topic of goat glands for what seemed like the fiftieth time:

Q: Haven't you stated that goat glands have "as a matter of cold sober fact, changed the color of patients' hair, smoothed the wrinkles out of their faces, and turned their complexions from a sickly pallor of old age and disease back to the ruddy glow of health"?

A: That is true.

Q: So explain to us please, how could you make that little testicle of a little—how old were the goats ordinarily?

A: About three weeks.

Q: That little testicle of a young goat, you claim that that lived and grew after you implanted it in a human testicle?

A: Some of them seemed to grow and enlarge and others, the majority of them, went through a process of absorption.

Q: Absorption?

A: Yes, sir, they were gradually absorbed. . . .

Q: You mean to say that little thing lived and was just like a part of the human testicle, and it was living in there after you put it in there?

A: No, sir, I don't conceive of it that way, I don't conceive of it as being a part of the human testicle. . . .

Q: You don't claim you connected up the nerves or any blood vessels?

A: Oh Lord, no.

Q: You just took this little thing separate and put it in that slit in the testicle and sewed it up?

A: Yes, sir.

Was it witness fatigue? Two days of captious questioning with his whole career at stake would have been enough to muddle anyone. But what he had just said—that the goat glands weren't grafted, just dumped in—was the precise opposite of what Brinkley had claimed for more than twenty years. It was the opposite of what he had said earlier the same day. Supporters could only look at him as if he'd lost his mind.

When the judge told him he was excused, Brinkley didn't hear at first.

52

As broadsides go, Brown's jury summation may not have matched the vitriolic grandeur achieved by London's solicitor general against that other fatally impetuous litigant, Oscar Wilde: an "appalling denunciation—like something out of Tacitus, like a passage in Dante, like one of Savonarola's indictments of the Popes of Rome." But it must have been impressive. Judge McMillan later told Clinton Brown (a former school chum) that it was "the best closing argument he had ever heard."

By a quirk of Texas law, it was also unrecorded. A snippet or two survives: "I want to win that five-hundred-dollar prize Dr. Brinkley is offering on the radio," Brown said at the end, "but I'll make a little change in the sentence. The sentence I offer in the contest is this: Dr. Brinkley is the foremost money-making surgeon in the world, *because* he had sense enough to know the weaknesses of human nature and gall enough to make a million dollars a year out of it."

How crusty Will Morriss Sr. tried to save his client is also unknown, but it mattered little by then. McMillan's charge to the jury came close to a directed verdict. While the judge explained that "the burden is upon the defendant, Dr. Morris Fishbein, to prove his defense, namely the substantial truth of the charges sued on," nevertheless "[t]here is no doubt that this plaintiff has been the subject of trouble in several places in this country. The question of his right to practice medicine has been raised several times. . . . It is manifest in his own and other evidence that this is not the first time an article of this kind has been written about him." McMillan listed damning facts for the jury to consider: "the revocation of Dr. Brinkley's license to practice medicine in Kansas, the revocation of his license in Connecticut in a general action against eclectic doctors, the refusal of California to grant him a permanent license, the cancellation of his broadcast privilege by the Federal Communications Commission and the revocation of a degree given him by a medical school in Italy," all of which were open to "fair and reasonable comment as a matter of public concern." Even if Dr. Fishbein had been "incorrect in certain particulars"—and the judge didn't suggest he was—such comments were "privileged and not to be considered libelous." Finally, McMillan pondered aloud over Brinkley's denunciation by the Kansas appeals court as an "empiric without moral sense." For reasons known only to himself the plaintiff had included every word of that truckload of insults in his own commissioned biography and, the judge said, ". . . the thing that occurs to me about it is that if a man feels he is capable of humiliation by virtue of an article of the character sued on here, then why would he in a book of his own copy a thing like that said about him and give it currency?" Someone who could libel himself that well didn't need any outside help.

The *Del Rio Evening News* had ballyhooed the trial with big headlines all week. On March 30 it reported the next development in a small column below the fold:

BRINKLEY WILL APPEAL CASE TO HIGHER COURT
Jury Returns Verdict Favoring Fishbein in Libel Suit

The jurors took four hours to find in favor of Dr. Fishbein: "that plaintiff should be considered a charlatan and quack in the ordinary, well-understood meaning of those words." Two things in particular had swayed them: the use of colored water that had bookended his career, and his twenty years of claiming that his goat-gland technique was a surgical graft. The evidence had buried Del Rio's favorite son.

When reporters turned to Fishbein for comment, he wasn't there: he was already in a cab speeding for the airport. Others caught him in Oklahoma City between planes. "If we can beat him there among his friends, we can beat him anywhere," the victor said, preparing to tuck into a big chicken dinner. Had he not been foolish enough to sue, Fishbein later added, Brinkley might have kept going for years.

The editor's old friend Arthur Cramp, forced into retirement by a heart attack in 1935, dropped him a note of congratulations: "[H]ow on earth did the AMA beat Brinkley on his own dunghill? I never would have believed it possible. If this keeps up I shall begin to develop some confidence in our courts!"

For the first time in his life, Brinkley avoided the press. He flew back to Little Rock in his Lockheed Electra monoplane from the Brinkley Hangar in Del Rio.

A few days later, a play called *The Man in Half Moon Street* opened in London. It was a Dorian Gray knockoff about a scientist who kills another man every ten years for his testicles, so he can implant them in himself and stay eternally young. "Leslie Banks is the scientist," an American reviewer wrote, "and so obviously believes in himself that we too are persuaded. He has a magnificently effective scene of pure theatre at the end, where his current set of glands wears out before its time, and he grows into an aged, aged man before our eyes."

What was once the salvation of mankind had turned into camp horror. It was the twilight of the glands.

In Ireland, Yeats died.

53

On December 14, 1939, Martin Luther King Jr. helped celebrate the premiere of *Gone With the Wind* dressed as a slave. The ten-year-old, along with the rest of the Ebenezer Baptist Choir of Atlanta, presented an evening of darky songs at the whites-only Junior League Ball, while not far away near Peachtree Street, the facade of Loew's Grand Theater was getting its last lick of paint. Complete with faux Greek columns, the exterior had been transformed into a replica of Tara, Scarlett O'Hara's beloved home.

The next night was thrill night. While spotlights raked the sky, an ocean of three hundred thousand people heaved against the soldiers lining both sides of the long red carpet. By the theater entrance, belles of Atlanta in hoop skirts and lace gloves, beaux in fawn-colored coats and breeches, young men in their grandfathers' uniforms complete with inconvenient swords, all milled about. Down every street in sight jutted a horizontal forest of Confederate flags. Take away the spotlights, and one might have thought that Grant had just surrendered at Appomattox.

At 7:30 they began to arrive—Selznick, Fleming, Mitchell, Leigh—and the night blazed with glamor, flashbulbs, and screaming. Stars large, medium, and small emerged from automobiles. Even some people with no connection to the movie got to walk down the red carpet. (*Who did they know?*) When Gable appeared, the soldiers had to link arms against the mob and fight to keep their footing.

It would have taken but a slight trick of the mind for Brinkley to believe it was all for him.

And for a moment or two it was. When their turn came, he escorted Minnie down the runway to the sort of nonspecific frenzy reserved for unidentified celebrities. Watching him go, a shrewd writer for the *Saturday Evening Post* saw a "jaunty-stepping, demurely paunchy, blond-goateed notable who might well have been mistaken for a Hollywood character actor specializing in physician roles."

In America the famous and the infamous are part of the same aristocracy. Perhaps this explains how Brinkley, just months after being stuffed and mounted in a federal courtroom in Del Rio, managed to snag a VIP invitation to the party of the decade. Could he possibly rebound yet again? The *Post* profile, which appeared the following April, talked up the apparent prosperity of the Little Rock venture—staff of thirty-five, two thousand letters a week—and seemed to treat his debacle in court as a mere detail. ("Despite fifteen years of concerted efforts by disgusted ill-wishers to get him off the air, Doctor, as his adherents call him, is still riding high.") Since the trial, Minnie said, her husband had received "five hundred thousand unsolicited letters" urging him to run for president.

Alas, Brinkley's front was as false as the Tara pasted on the outside of Loew's. Just as Fishbein had predicted, being officially branded a fraud by a judge and jury unleashed a slew of lawsuits against the goat-gland king. A lawyer in Little Rock wrote Fishbein that his client was pursuing Brinkley for $602,500, on the grounds that he "has rendered our client sterile, impotent and has totally disabled him." Another complaint charged "criminal negligence in permitting a patient to bleed to death on the operating table." At the time of the *Gone With the Wind* premiere, the newly crowned "board-certified quack" faced suits of more than $3 million and counting—this despite his new policy of giving refunds if the patient died. Even his business manager in Little Rock sued him for malpractice.

Meanwhile the IRS, with its infallible nose for carrion, was coming after him for back taxes.

"I have paid nothing towards fixing up the Country Club Hospital and I am in debt clear up to my eyes," Brinkley wrote one of his staff physicians in June 1940. "I have had to lay off a lot of employees, have had to reduce the salaries of Doctors, Nurses and office help, almost in half and I have been in worse circumstances here in this state than I have ever been in my life."

Attempting to have the verdict overturned, he gave the court of appeals the chance to reinsult him. The Supreme Court denied review. Yet all the while promotional literature kept whirling out of his Dupligraph.

"Dear Friend: You failed to save $25.00 during January. You failed to save $22.50 during February. Will you fail to save $20.00 during March? Each month the amount you can save grows less. . . ."

A petition signed by twenty-four of Del Rio's leading citizens implored Dr. and Mrs. Brinkley to relocate their hospital back there, "where full confidence in them prevails and they are respected and loved." Brinkley was amenable, but with creditors and claimants on him like the Furies he couldn't make the shift, at least until he reversed his disastrous cash flow.

Many thought the doctor would make a bold move. Few thought it would involve the Dilley Aircraft School.

With the lava of war spreading across Europe, and American involvement probable, the world needed heroes. It also needed a place where the craven and selfish could go till it was all over, and that was what Brinkley alertly hoped to provide. No one had looked out for him like this when he was trying to beat the draft. And you couldn't ask for more motivated spenders.

"Why squads right and squads left at $21 per month when you can get a good paying job as an aviation mechanic? . . . [You] must decide whether you are to dig ditches [and] carry a gun or be a trained mechanic away from the bullets. . . . Thousands of jobs are going begging. . . . Our students are taken before they can complete the courses. . . ."

Before he took over, the Dilley School was a modest shop in Kansas City with courses in welding and airplane mechanics. Many ads and spurious endorsements later, the doctor had drawn scores of applicants. The big attraction was that Dilley graduates couldn't be drafted.

Or so he claimed. That he even tried to get away with a lie that big was cause for mystified comment when the Better Business Bureau took him to court. In less than a year the school was in receivership and Brinkley charged with looting the corporation.

By December 1940, Minnie was so frazzled she had to get away for a while. She fled to a place she had once been happy. "Nassau is beautiful," she wrote a friend, "like a white pearl in a Turquoise mounting. . . . I did see the Windsors. She looks bad and pitiful, he is little and cute and sure is gay. . . ."

When he declared bankruptcy in San Antonio early in 1941, Dr. Brinkley listed more than $300,000 in assets and more than $1 million in debts. If the records were sketchier than courts like to see, there was good reason for it. "I never had any books," he explained.

Not that he and Minnie were out on the street. Bankruptcy law protected their mansion, furnishings, clothes, diamonds, insurance policies, photographs of the doctor, and one car. And as his creditors soon discovered, he tried to keep everything else, a task to which he brought a well of cunning and ingenuity. Even before he reached court he shifted assets to Minnie, Johnny Boy, and various friends. "This was the beginning," a journalist wrote, "of an exciting game of hare and hounds played for more than one and a half million dollars. . . ."

On March 24, with Mrs. Brinkley now a bankrupt, too, distressed creditors swarmed the federal courthouse in Del Rio to press their claims. Fingering his largest diamond ring, the doctor affably told the judge that while he couldn't say precisely where most of his money had gone, he could offer the gentlemen present a partial settlement— six horses, ninety head of cattle, forty ducks, and a harpoon gun—to be divided loaves-and-fishes-style among them. Slight mining interests and real estate might yield something, too, but unfortunately the radio station belonged to the Mexican government, the hospital had not been incorporated under his name. . . .

The shell game to protect his wealth ultimately failed. After that he was dead but he wouldn't lie down. He began studying to become an ordained minister by mail and, after consulting an astrologer, filed an application with the Texas secretary of state to run for the U.S. Senate. "I am bankrupt and have no money to contribute to my campaign," he announced. "If I am elected, it must be a free-will offering from the people of Texas who love and trust me." The offering was unforthcoming, and he soon withdrew.

Worse, far worse, Mexico and the United States ended their long feud and reached agreement on allocating bandwidths. Brinkley's ouster was part of the deal. When Mexican troops seized and sacked XERA in the summer of 1941, an AP reporter telegraphed that the station was accused of transmitting "news broadcasts unsuitable to new world" under the aegis of "foreigners sympathetic to Nazi cause." Along the border there were rumors that Brinkley was a Nazi spy.

Still, it was not till July 21, when he wrote his wife from Kansas City, that he finally acknowledged all was lost:

> Honey,
>   It seems my heart will break since you phoned XERA was being torn down. As long as this did not happen I had a faint hope. . . .
>   My health is gone. I am ready for the bed and out. . . .
>   Love, Daddy

Three days later he had a heart attack.

54

W hen Dr. Brinkley was stricken in Kansas City," Minnie remembered, "Father Flanagan came by plane and sat all day by his bedside." Otherwise friends were few and far between, and Minnie, bitter in her ruin, knew exactly whom to blame. To an unknown correspondent she wrote: "The American Medical Association framed Dr. Brinkley. . . . Dr. Fishbein caused all the trouble. . . ."

In a Kansas City hospital, Brinkley's health crumbled. When a blood clot formed in late August, his left leg had to be amputated. A couple of weeks later the U.S. Post Office Department, rising from two decades of zombie sleep, charged him with mail fraud. A federal marshal appeared at his bedside with a warrant containing a fifteen-count indictment, including the vague but humiliating charge that he "did falsely pretend that John R. Brinkley was a great surgeon, scientist and physician."

"Well," Brinkley said as he took the paper, "I guess there isn't any danger of my running away."

Since he was too weak to leave his bed, prosecutors postponed the trial, but they arrested Minnie for mail fraud, too. On January 10, 1942, the doctor wrote one of his attorneys, Wallace Davis of San Antonio, begging for help:

> I am in bankruptcy and everything I owned has been
> sold. . . .

I have been in bed since August 23rd. My weight fell
from 175 to 130. The amputated bone is diseased and the
leg has never healed properly. I am in constant pain. . . .

Until we were indicted we could borrow money, but
since the indictment even our personal friends will not
take a chance. . . .

In days gone by I paid you every cent you charged
me. One time I had to borrow the money to pay you,
but you were paid. I am flat on my back and helpless
and I am asking for a little mercy. . . .

Believing correctly that Davis would ignore his plea, Minnie
appealed to a friend of her own, Maury Hughes.

"If this case comes to trial we are sunk. . . . We have no money to
get the necessary witnesses and employ local counsel. . . . I do not
want you to labor under the impression that so many do that if we
have to we will dig up the money some place. It is this very thought in
the minds of so many that we have money hid away in an old tin can
that blocks our progress. . . .

"I would to God that I could have you understand this situation
like we know it. If you are going to save us from destruction you must
do it alone and on your own efforts."

The doctor did have one bright moment toward the end. He
learned that Norman Baker had been convicted of mail fraud, a
cancer cure consisting of watermelon seed, corn silk, carbolic acid,
and water being deemed insufficient to save him from four years in
Leavenworth. Brinkley (fallaciously) claimed credit for Baker's fall. "I
got my friends in Arkansas to crack down on him," he said, sitting up
in bed. "The D.A., the judge and I sat around and decided how much
to give him on the mail charge. . . . I guess I've paid him back for
pinching my patients and that fifteen hundred dollars."

But it was a brief respite. On May 6, he sent Minnie a Mother's
Day message in an elegiac key.

"We are being tried in the fires of persecution and disappointment. . . . We must stand together, walk side by side and look to a glorious eternity. If I cross the bar before you I will be waiting and watching for you. . . .

"You have a responsibility to our son John. . . . Lend your time and talents to him. He is a delicate flower like his father."

Later Minnie attached her own note to this:

Last Love Letter
   Our love was true and our Loyalty made for Success

When he died in his sleep in San Antonio on May 26, 1942, Brinkley was one of the most famous people in the United States, and one who had just escaped multiple prosecutions. He was eulogized in Del Rio and buried under a large monument in Memphis, Tennessee, the city where he and Minnie had met.

After his long reign, capped by a downfall of Shakespearean economy, he received the tributes from enemies customary at the close. "What a little tinkering with his character might have done," said William Allen White. "[A] little more honesty here, a little more intelligence there . . . would have made him a really great leader of men." Morris Fishbein offered a salute of sorts: "The centuries to come may never produce again such blatancy, such fertility of imagination, and such ego." But nobody caught the moment like an anonymous geezer in the crowd: "I knowed he was bilking me, but . . . I liked him anyway."

The doctor died richer than he knew.

Epilogue

mbrose Bierce defined a quack as "a murderer without a license," but given the Jurassic state of malpractice laws in Brinkley's day, a license to kill was just what he had. He made the most of it, too: though perhaps not the worst serial killer in American history, ranked by body count alone he is at least a finalist for the crown. At the Kansas medical-board hearing in 1930, roughly the midpoint of his career, prosecutors proved that at least forty-two people (some of whom weren't sick to start with) had entered his clinic vertical and departed horizontal, to say nothing of the others like housepainter John Homback who staggered off and collapsed somewhere else. Add to them the ten years' worth of patients still to come, and the blind ravages of *Medical Question Box,* and you have slaughter on a scale the worst midnight maniac never approaches. His career was sustained in part by America's deep reluctance to criminalize greed. Not until 1964 did the country's first bungling doctor go to jail for murdering a patient, and by then the mortiferous Milford Messiah was long gone from the scene.

Bringing this deathmonger to heel the only way he could, Fishbein did more than just stop one quack. He won for the AMA the undisputed authority to set licensing standards for doctors nationwide. The case marked the boundary line between the unregulated melee that was American medicine going back two or three centuries, and the sober centralization that has defined it since. The benefits of this change have not been entirely unalloyed. That vampire's instinct which keeps power always thirsting for more power has often marked the AMA, leading, for example, to its conviction in the Sherman antitrust case in the early 1940s. (The organization paid a fine; Fishbein himself wasn't penalized.) On the other hand, thanks to the association's dominance, it's more likely today that your doctor's diploma came from a real school.

Fishbein plied his harpoon in many waters, but Brinkley was his Moby Dick. Forced from his post in 1949 by AMA members tired of his blotting out the sun, the ex-editor went on writing and lecturing at the same breathless pace till shortly before his death on September 27, 1976. Earlier that year, alertly responding to two centuries of complaints, Congress had at last passed the Medical Device Amendments to the Pure Food and Drug Act—the laws banning quack gadgetry—for which he had so long crusaded.

At Fishbein's funeral Chicago's mayor Richard J. Daley eulogized him, as did a host of luminaries in his field. Today at the University of Chicago, the Morris Fishbein Center for the History of Science and Medicine perpetuates his name. In general, however, the fireball editor has suffered the fate of most crime busters: the Brinkley triumph aside, most of what he accomplished has not endured. Since his death new quacks with new quackeries have sprouted faster than ever; whatever ground he cleared the jungle soon reclaimed. Today bogus cancer and weight-loss treatments, biological dentistry, ear candling (putting a candle in your ear), Wild Yam Cream, chelation therapy, Qigong, and untold thousands of other get-well-quick schemes keep their inventors swimming in champagne.

But John Brinkley's legacy has been wide and deep.

Like Bogart, the doctor was misinformed. XERA wasn't torn down; it was rescued by two of his former employees, who aside from toning down the quack part didn't change a thing. "Hank Snow, Ernest Tubb, Lefty Frizzell, Hank Williams, Jimmie Davis, Pee Wee King—most everybody who was anybody . . . paid a visit to Ciudad to spin some discs and tell some tales," a staffer from that era recalled. Sadly, few of the records they cut at the station survive. "They became very popular in Mexico, these old platters," said

Brinkley's station manager, Don Howard. ". . . They made wonderful shingles if you [were] putting them on a roof because they were this acetate outside and aluminum inside and they'd last forever."

By then Brinkley's innovations—replacing live music with recordings, broadcasting long-distance via telephone, even the AM format itself—were taking hold throughout the industry. And still Del Rio stayed in the picture. There was music in the cafés at night and revolution in the air well into the 1950s, especially when the doc's old seat at the microphone passed to Bob Smith of Brooklyn, New York. To the Japanese he was the "Emperor of Pleasing Graciousness," to the Germans the "Laughing Chancellor of Comedy." But Americans knew him as Wolfman Jack.

The great Señor Wolfman found XERA (now XERF) pretty much the same old playpen. "All you had to do was file one form sheet," he said, "run the National Hour every Sunday night, and pay your taxes, and the Mexicans would let you do whatever the hell you wanted." For a while on the air as a sort of homage to Brinkley he peddled jars of pellets called Florex. ("You know, maybe the marriage is getting a little stale in the naughty department. Well, one of these pills in mama's orange juice . . .") More important, he was Brinkley's spiritual disciple, making history by giving the world an earful of the unexpected: "We gonna rock your soul with a steady roll and pay our dues with the BLUES!"

It started with "the Chess sound" out of Chicago—records by Muddy Waters, Howlin' Wolf, Little Walter—and exploded from there. Across the continent Wolfman Jack, Fat Daddy Washington, Magnificent Montague, and other border-blaster DJs of the new generation spread the music that mainstream American radio tried to wish away: hard-core blues and R & B, Clyde McPhatter, Hank Ballard, Joe Turner, the Platters, the Clovers . . .

"Get naked, blow the evil weed, and kiss your teachers!"

Black music got its first nationwide kick in the pants from the border blasters, just like hillbilly music before it. The tangled voodoo of country and blues these stations now carried ("an all-American music that transcended format and ranged from Hank Williams to the hard-core funk of James Brown") overwhelmed the plastic pop machine and revolutionized the musical tastes of America's new generation. The blasters spawned the white-black crossover culture, fueling the rise of rock and roll, and that paved the way for—well, you name it.

In the 1980s Mexico's border blasters faded out, overtaken by time and technology. But another Brinkley legacy yet survives there: quack clinics, especially "cancer-cure" retreats, still lurk just outside the reach of U.S. law. For decades rough signs—SANDWICHES LAETRILE FOOD—have pointed the desperate toward clinics in Tijuana and elsewhere. Movie star Steve McQueen died of lung cancer on a last-ditch visit to a healer in Juarez.

It took Hitler invading Poland to get the world's mind off glands. In later years Dr. Serge Voronoff, according to one acquaintance, "lived to be ridiculed, but bore it with dignity" until his death in 1951. A close friend, however, described him as deeply depressed late in life, "troubled by the fact that nobody seemed to be following in his footsteps." Worse, some of his two thousand transplants were coming back to haunt him. He was shattered to learn that his monkey glands had given some patients syphilis.

His great rival, Dr. Eugen Steinach, fared better. On his eightieth birthday the *New York Times* called his research "distinguished by its thoroughness and originality. He was probably the most powerful influence in leading the new knowledge of sex hormones into the proper channel"—e.g., the synthesizing of testosterone—"though his operation had lost its vogue." In other words, his errors and failures had suggested better paths to others. That's science.

Still, the constituency for truth is always finite, especially in the youth-recovery game. After the Second World War, Dr. Paul Niehans of Switzerland inherited the mantle of "rejuvenator to the stars." ("I was able to watch both Steinach and Voronoff perform," he said, "and so profited from their mistakes.") At his Clinique La Prairie on

Lake Geneva, Niehans provided "cellular therapy" to wizened celebrities like Somerset Maugham, Konrad Adenauer, Georges Braque, and Pope Pius XII. As *Look* magazine ("Is This Man Keeping the Pope Alive?") explained the technique in 1957: "When an organ ails, 'fresh cells' are procured from the corresponding part of the foetus of an animal or from a very young calf, ewe or pig. The cells are mashed into a solution which is injected directly into the patient's body. . . ." Professor Brown-Sequard at least had shown great staying power.

Today rejuvenation is a global bazaar of infomercials and Web addresses, tools and toys for every need. For men, the anxious quest for good pole position continues, whether it be with Viagra or Chinese Crocodile Penis Pills "made from a 2,000-year-old recipe." Steroids, a more specialized male fetish, are a popular devil's bargain. Women, on the other hand, though not immune to the lure of muscle mass, ordinarily fret more about packaging than performance. Eyelash transplants have been with us since the 1970s, but the past few years have seen an explosion in cosmetic surgery blind to reason and risk. In 2001 a form of bovine collagen was blamed for an outbreak of Creutzfeldt-Jakob syndrome, a potentially lethal disorder linked to mad cow disease, yet this did nothing to slow the stampede for fuller lips and smoother skin. "Most women would find the prospect of dying wrinkled a lot worse than the prospect of dying of dementia from collagen," observed Richard G. Glogau, a San Francisco dermatologist. "As long as they don't drop dead thirty seconds later, they'll do it." Certainly nips and tucks can sometimes promote self-esteem. It's equally true that the pop-eyed and pole-necked look can send the same message as a man in a bad toupee.

That's one reason others have scorned these surface tokens of youthiness in order to pursue "practical immortality," a movement devoted like the gland craze of yore to beating back time itself. As rejuvenation guru Dr. Ronald Klatz has put it, "We're not about growing old gracefully. We're about never growing old." Places like the Palm Springs Life Extension Institute and the International

Longevity Center of New York regard aging not as a natural process but as a disease. And the cure? Till the ultimate youth pill comes along (the Holy Grail in pharmaceutical research), some no-age prophets have been promoting hGH, or human growth hormone, a nonsteroid defined as a "polypeptide hormone synthesized and secreted by the anterior pituitary gland." Yes, glands are back as a $1.5 to $2 billion–a–year business promising "glowing skin, increased muscle mass, elevated sex drive, a lighter mood, sharper mental acuity and the whiz-bang metabolism of an 18-year-old." It's not immortality, but it's not bad—if one discounts the risks, claimed by some, of cancer and premature death.

Some scientists, more rigorous perhaps, hope to stop time by changing the makeup of our cells. At a millennial gathering of the Society for Regenerative Medicine, Cynthia Kenyon, a University of California molecular biologist, reported on efforts to identify the "grim-reaper gene" and "fountain of youth gene," and predicted much-expanded life spans in the twenty-first century. Michael West of Advanced Cell Technology added: "We are close to transferring the immortal characteristics of germ cells to our bodies and essentially eliminating aging." According to a 2005 issue of *Harvard Magazine* ("Is Aging Necessary?"), scientists working with yeast, roundworms, and fruit flies "have found that they can dramatically extend life span by tweaking single genes. The altered organisms don't just live longer, they age more slowly, in many cases retaining youthful characteristics even after normal individuals have died." Still, even a very old fruit fly is gone before you know it.

What's left? Cloning is still out of reach. An optimist might join poor Ted Williams hanging upside down in a nitrogen-filled tank in Arizona. Futurist Ray Kurzweil predicts that computer hardware will be powerful enough to run a functional model of the human mind by the 2020s, which would open the door to something called "mind uploading," or "the transfer of the human mind/consciousness to a more durable material vessel." This would allow you, or a very detailed map of you, to live on in your laptop.

But all these outlandish choices may soon be moot. In the fall of 2006 researchers at the National Institute of Aging and Harvard Medical School reported on the supercharged potential of a substance found in red wine, known as resveratrol. Giving megadoses to mice dramatically increased not only their life span but their endurance as well. Even on artery-clogging diets, their heart rates dropped, and they could run twice as far on a treadmill. In short, resveratrol "makes you look like a trained athlete without the training," a French researcher said. Dr. Leonard Guarente, biology professor at MIT, called it "an entirely new therapeutic strategy to address the diseases of aging."

If practical immortality turns out to be as close as the nearest liquor store, we can only salute the prescience of Benjamin Franklin a dozen lifetimes ago: "I wish it were possible to invent a method of embalming drowned persons, in such a manner that they may be recalled to life at any period, however distant; for having a very ardent desire to see and observe the state of America a hundred years hence, I should prefer to any ordinary death, the being immersed in a cask of Madeira wine, with a few friends, till that time, to be then recalled to life by the solar warmth of my dear country."

After her own mail-fraud conviction, for which she got probation, Minnie Brinkley lived on in the Del Rio mansion for the next three decades. Stucco cracked, weeds grew. There was talk that she entertained a string of young men, but nobody held it against her. In 1962, when Milford was about to be swallowed by a dam, she tried to get permission to post a lighted buoy on the site of the old Brinkley Hospital.

"[My husband was] forty-five years ahead of his time," Minnie told a visitor when organ transplants first made news. "They said at the time that no foreign body could live inside a human, and just look what they're doing now!" She confided that goat-gland transplants were still being done in secret: "They're just not being advertised. But the operation was too good to throw away."

And when she died in 1978, she was borne to glory on the crashing power chords of ZZ Top:

> *Do you remember*
> *back in 1966?*
> *Country Jesus, hillbilly blues,*
> *that's where I learned my licks.*
> *Oh, from coast to coast and line to line,*
> *in every county there,*
> *I'm talkin' 'bout that outlaw X*
> *is cuttin' through the air. . . .*
>
> *We can all thank Doctor B*
> *who stepped across the line.*
> *With lots of watts he took control,*
> *the first one of its kind.*
> *So listen to your radio*
> *most each and every night*
> *'Cause if you don't, I'm sure you won't*
> *get to feeling right.*
>
> *. . . I heard it, I heard it,*
> *I heard it on the X.*

Acknowledgments

There's a joke well known among writers, the punch line of which is "My agent came to my house?" David Black has never actually been to my house, but his involvement in my career, and in particular this endeavor, has transformed both. Another client once called him a "proposal Nazi"; six drafts and a year's work later I knew why and was grateful for it. (A proposal overseen by David has an unanswerable solidity, like the pyramids.) Throughout he has been generous with his support, moral and otherwise. Moreover, it was his question ("Who's Morris Fishbein?") that made the whole project snap into place.

I feel very fortunate to have landed with Rick Horgan at Crown. Some arranged marriages of editors and writers are more successful than others. This one worked. With his shrewd eye and gentle insistence, he has pulled a better book out of me than I realized was there.

My great gratitude to the research staff at the Chappaqua library for handling dozens of arcane requests with diligence, imagination, and good humor. Carolyn Resnick, Martha Alcott, Michele Capozella, Maryanne Eaton, Paula Peyraud, Cathy Paulsen, Chris Trzcinski, Shelby Monroe, Vicky Fugua: if you quailed when you saw me coming, you never showed it. I couldn't have written this book without your help.

A host of other librarians and archivists aided me along the way: Lin Fredericksen and Christie Stanley at the Kansas State Historical Society; Robert Tenuta and Andrea Bainbridge at the AMA archives in Chicago; Shirley Miller and Robin Heppner at the Escanaba Public

Library; Sandy Roscoe at the Special Collections Research Center, University of Chicago; Lee Lincoln at the Whitehead Memorial Museum in Del Rio; Willie Braudaway and the staff of the Val Verde County Library; Debbie Speer of the Historic Greenville Foundation and Cori Dulmage at the Greenville County Library; Debbie Vaughan at the Chicago Historical Society; Arlene Shaner at the New York Academy of Medicine Library; George Frizell at the Western Carolina University Library; and Rita Forrester and Fred Boyd of the Carter Family Foundation. To all, my sincere appreciation.

Special thanks to Justin Fishbein, one of the few living links to this story, who was a great help across many months; to Janette Carter for sharing her memories of Brinkley; and to Louise Faulkner, widow of Roy, the least lonesome cowboy of the 1930s.

To Richard Duggin, Jenna Lucas, and all my fellow misfits at the University of Nebraska MFA writing program (the gold standard in low-res), thanks for all your support, even though you have left me confused as to the difference between work and play.

My thanks to Laurence Senelick for his erudite contributions and for a grand forty years (yikes) of friendship, as well as to Jeff and Judi Seal, Tom and Terry Allen, and Ellen Stern, for help above and beyond. Also to Julian Pavia for his zeal and attention to detail, to Mary Jane Brock, Susan Adams, Lee Aitken, Wendy Martin, Susan Raihofer, Leigh Ann Eliseo, Pat Larkin, Jeannie Zusy, Patricia Lear, Dr. Molly O'Neill, Anna Monardo, Dr. Bob Greenspan, and as always to Doris Betts for setting me on my way.

Finally, my family and I want to express our immense gratitude to the whole Roaring Brook School community in Chappaqua, and especially to our Pine Cliff neighbors and to Steffi Green and her sisters of mercy. Who knew lasagna could mean so much?

Notes

Key to archive sources:
JRB papers, KSHS = John R. Brinkley papers, Kansas State Historical Society, Topeka, Kansas
Carson papers, KSHS = Gerald Carson papers, Kansas State Historical Society
MF papers, U. of Chi = Morris Fishbein papers, Special Collections, University of Chicago Research Center
MB papers, WMM = Minnie Brinkley papers, Whitehead Memorial Museum, Del Rio, Texas

Prologue

1 *Under the Knife:* Drawn primarily from press coverage in the *Kansas City Star,* the *Kansas City Journal-Post,* and the *Topeka Daily Capital;* also Carson, *Roguish World.*

Chapter 1

6 Many of the Reinhardts' exploits are detailed in Holbrook, *Golden Age of Quackery.* See also Anderson, *Snake Oil.*

9 *known as a Quaker doctor:* Lee, *Bizarre Careers;* Carson, *Roguish World.* The origins of the Quaker doctor are from Anderson, *Snake Oil.*

11 *"Any one, male or female":* Young, *The Toadstool Millionaires.*

11 *Dr. Benjamin Rush:* For more on Benjamin Rush's career as "Doctor Doom," see Armstrong and Armstrong, *The Great American Medicine Show.*

12 *came along with his "galvanic tractors":* At one time the luckless Washington was also a patient of Dr. Perkins.

Chapter 2

13 *"incredibly long lanes of street-lamps":* Lewis and Smith, *Chicago.*

13 The portrait of the city's moneyed class is drawn chiefly from Longstreet, *Chicago.*

14 *Orchis Extract* and *Armour*: Bullough, *Science in the Bedroom*.
14 *"the disastrous appearance of those patients"*: Morris Fishbein, *An Autobiography*.
16 *"always pitying himself to gain confidence"*: Sally Wike Engren, letter to *The Pink Rag*, October 11, 1932, AMA files.
17 Chief source on the Brevoort Hotel: Chicago Historical Society.

Chapter 3

19 The story of Brinkley and Crawford's Electro Medic escapade is based on contemporary coverage in the *Greenville (South Carolina) Daily News*; *JAMA*, January 1928; James Crawford deposition (in *District Court of Geary County, State of Kansas, John R. Brinkley, Plaintiff* v. *Morris Fishbein and William S. Yates, Defendants,* October 8, 1930); Carson, *Roguish World*. See also C. A. David, *Greenville of Old*.

Chapter 4

23 Fishbein's early professional career: Fishbein, *An Autobiography*.
23 *"because I have so much to say"*: Arthur J. Snider, draft of Morris Fishbein profile for *Medical World News*, 1964, MF papers, U. of Chi.
23 *Arthur Cramp*: Young, *Medical Messiahs*.
25 *"vague, obliging and long defunct"*: As quoted in Carson, *Roguish World*.
25 *as if on an urgent call*: Wardlaw, "The Goat-Gland Man."
25 *"physician and clerk"*: Rensler, Ph.D. dissertation.
25 *"considerable lubricity"*: John R. Brinkley as quoted by Morris Fishbein, "Quackery in American Medicine," *Bulletin of the Los Angeles County Medical Association,* August 16, 1962.
25 Spondylotherapy: Young, *Medical Messiahs*. See also Armstrong and Armstrong, *The Great American Medicine Show*. As Dr. Abrams once wrote with striking candor, "The physician is only allowed to think he knows it all, but the quack, ungoverned by conscience, is permitted to know he knows it all; and with a fertile mental field for humbuggery, truth can never successfully compete with untruth."

Chapter 5

27 *"I did the work"*: Chase, *Sound and Fury*.
28 *"rectal fistula, multiple"*: Carson, *Roguish World*.
28 *On the edge of town*: Fowler and Crawford, *Border Radio*.
28 *"as I should urgently advise"*: Carson, *Roguish World*.
30 *"I have a scheme"*: Lee, *Bizarre Careers*.

Chapter 6

31 *"it was the custom"*: New York Times, April 23, 1925.

31 *The notion of priming one's privates*: Herman, "Rejuvenation."

32 *"Incantation for Transforming"*: New York Times, March 24, 1925; November 10, 1925.

32 *an herb called satyrion*: Theophrastus claimed that the herb would enable a man to perform seventy consecutive acts of sexual intercourse.

32 *Mars was fit for human habitation*: Topeka Daily State Journal, October 11, 1930.

33 *the snoligostus, the ogopogo*: MacDougall, *Hoaxes*.

33 Brown-Sequard's career is based on contemporary newspaper coverage; Trimmer, *Rejuvenation*; and other sources. For a good thumbnail survey of the European gland movement, see Schulteiss, Denil, and Jonas, "Rejuvenation in the Early 20th Century."

35 *"We chatted a moment"*: Fishbein, *An Autobiography*.

35 *"and could even understand a joke"*: Carson, *Roguish World*.

36 *giving prisoners nose jobs*: Hallinan, *Going Up the River*.

37 *"I dare assert . . . that the monkey"*: For more on Voronoff's career, see Friedman, *A Mind of Its Own*; McGrady, *The Youth Doctors*.

38 *"raised the platform of efficiency"*: Steinach as quoted in McGrady, *The Youth Doctors*.

38 *"Does any scientific discovery"*: Brinkley aside, the other great gland stars wholly believed in what they were doing. "Although these procedures seem bizarre today, the fact that Steinach and Voronoff reported many 'cures' before these methods succumbed to medical progress does not necessarily place them among the quacks of their era. On the contrary, their treatments, like those of Brown-Sequard, show how similar the therapeutic results of unconscious error and conscious fraud can be" (Hoberman, *Testosterone Dreams*).

Chapter 7

39 *"He saved us"*: Lee, *Bizarre Careers*.

40 *"the testes of a goat"*: Shah, "Erectile Dysfunction Through the Ages."

41 *"stupid types"*: S. Rodriguez, "Goat Glands Brinkley," *Lust Magazine* online.

42 *"She seemed to hobble along"*: Brinkley file, AMA archives.

42 *"If Mrs. Brinkley lived near you"*: Carson, *Roguish World*.

43 *eye-opening aroma*: Fowler and Crawford, *Border Radio*; Lee, *Bizarre Careers*.

43 *"old fools"*: Ex-nurse Louise Ferris, as quoted in the *Kansas City Star*, April 5, 1930.

44 *"By God, we've got it!"*: Lee, *Bizarre Careers*.

44 *"This is to certify . . . Ex-Lax every month"*: Young, *Toadstool Millionaires*.

Chapter 8

45 Thorek's encounter with Lydston: Thorek, *A Surgeon's World.*

45 *the first monkey-to-man testicle transplant:* Within two years, Voronoff would be claiming it was possible to "transplant all the vital organs of a chimpanzee to human beings." *New York Times,* June 20, 1922.

45 *Lydston believed that Voronoff:* Others agreed. In an otherwise laudatory review of Voronoff's book *Life* and his "great discovery," the *New York Times* (November 7, 1920) complained that he had not given sufficient credit to Lydston's work.

46 *"Oh, zat is fine!":* Carson, *Roguish World.*

47 *"Dr. J. R. Brinkley Swamped":* Chicago Herald and Examiner, February 8, 1920.

48 *"the most gullible of all":* Thus allowing the quack to enjoy "the supreme pleasure of despising the intellect" (de Francesco, *The Power of the Charlatan*).

49 *The hosannas of the law-school administrator:* Lee, *Bizarre Careers.* Tobias was the perfect combination of reputable and zany. Pivotal to Brinkley's career, his case (aside from Stittsworth's) received more coverage than any other.

49 *"These operations will increase the birth rate":* Chicago Tribune, February 16, 1920.

49 *"Was the ancient mystery":* Thorek, *A Surgeon's World.*

Chapter 9

50 *"At this moment I cannot":* New Haven Courier, July 13, 1921.

50 *Now an Arkansas supplier:* Chase, *Sound and Fury.*

51 *"You must get yourself so organized":* Letter from Brinkley to Osborn, n.d., JRB papers, KSHS.

51 *"never thought talking to people":* Lee, *Bizarre Careers.*

51 *The high whine of energy:* At home, housekeeper Arfie Cordray remembered, Minnie Brinkley's tongue was "loose at both ends," but the doctor was usually reading "a book or something."

51 Brinkley's violent outbursts: Carson, *Roguish World.*

51 *"Christ did not build the Milford Church":* Chicago Tribune, August 17, 1930. See also Lee, *Bizarre Careers.*

52 *"You are possessed with power":* Carson, *Roguish World.*

52 *"[Brinkley] asked me how I was getting along":* Lee, *Bizarre Careers.*

53 *"I suppose a goat gland":* Zwonitzer and Hirshberg, *Will You Miss Me When I'm Gone?*

53 *Stories had surfaced over the past year:* For example, "TWO MORE LOSE GLANDS . . . Search for Knife Men," *Los Angeles Times,* October 15, 1922, page 1.

53 *"You are able to pay":* Kansas City Star, July 16, 1930.

55 *Brinkley's assistant, Dr. Osborn:* Carson, *Roguish World.*

Chapter 10

56   *"If the operation is a success"*: As quoted in Chase, *Sound and Fury.*

56   *"any wizard, geomancer, soothsayer"*: Morrow, *Los Angeles, City of Dreams.* Other material in this chapter is drawn from Wright, "Los Angeles—the Chemically Pure"; Louis Adamic and Aldous Huxley in Ulin, *Writing Los Angeles.*

58   Chandler's life and exploits are drawn primarily from Gottlieb, *Thinking Big,* and McDougal, *Privileged Son.*

58   *His newspaper, most agreed, was lousy:* To put it mildly. "The L.A. *Times* was venal, vicious, stupid, and dull. It was abominably written and poorly edited. It existed to advance the unfathomably reactionary political views of the family that controlled it" (Hendrik Hertzberg, *The New Yorker,* April 23 and 30, 2001).

59   *"Laboratory analysis shows"*: *Los Angeles Times,* March 6, 1922.

59   *"the swelling of the body"*: As quoted in Fowler and Crawford, *Border Radio.*

61   *"along the lines of the Battle Creek health resort"*: *Los Angeles Times,* June 19, 1922.

Chapter 11

62   *"Fishbein is a wonder!"*: As quoted in Lingeman, *Sinclair Lewis.*

63   *Fishbein's particular passion was the theater:* Fishbein, *An Autobiography.*

63   *Through Fishbein, Lewis got a taste:* See Drury, *Dining in Chicago,* and Hecht, *Child of the Century.* Sinclair Lewis was only one of many guests the "round table" welcomed over the years, including D. W. Griffith, Ed Wynn, Ford Madox Ford, and the Marx Brothers.

64   *"full of tremendous whoops"*: As quoted in Rascoe, *Before I Forget.*

64   *"a medical savant"*: Hecht, *Child of the Century.*

64   *He improvised playlets:* Rascoe, *Before I Forget.*

65   Lindlahr's methods and the workings of his sanitarium are drawn primarily from AMA archives. Fishbein spent a chapter eviscerating naturopathy in his book *Fads and Quackery in Healing* (1932).

66   *"Do we want some reviewer"*: Sandburg's wife, Paula, later won awards as a goat breeder after becoming convinced that goat's milk had cured her gallbladder problems.

Chapter 12

67   *"Criminality Is Cured"*: *Los Angeles Times,* November 12, 1922, front page.

68   *"The harder they hit me"*: See, for example, *Syracuse Herald,* July 9, 1933. It was a line he returned to throughout his career.

68   *Avon Foreman:* Time-Life, *This Fabulous Century, 1920–1930.*

68 *"It is modern throughout"*: Promotional material, JRB papers, KSHS.

69 *"My Dear Friend"*: Brinkley form letter, October 25, 1922, JRB papers, KSHS.

70 *"two of the finest people"*: Printed testimonial dated September 14, 1922 (AMA files). A year and a half later the senator was dead.

70 *"the reading public has become"*: New York Times, June 4, 1922.

72 *tapping into the doctor's line*: Casey, More Interesting People.

72 *"Under the spreading chestnut tree"*: Friedman, A Mind of Its Own.

73 *Brinkley had this angle covered*: Lee, Bizarre Careers.

74 *"blood marriage"*: New York Times, May 20, 1925.

Chapter 13

75 *"a national enthusiast [who]"*: Mencken, My Life as Author and Editor.

76 *"Gene really is a Christ spirit"*: As quoted in Lingeman, Sinclair Lewis.

77 *"Here now in the door"*: Versions of that night's subsequent adventures appear in Fishbein, An Autobiography; DeKruif, The Sweeping Wind; Schorer, Sinclair Lewis.

Chapter 14

81 *"no evidence of curving"*: Chase, Sound and Fury.

81 *After that, journeying south*: Carson, Roguish World.

82 *"it is now possible to control"*: Bernays, Propaganda.

82 *Maharajah Thakou Galub of Morvi*: Minneapolis News, September 17, 1921.

83 *"The children of parents who have been endowed"*: Ballou, "Gland Transplantation Is Link in Chain of Scientific Progress." A man of catholic interests, Ballou was listed in Who's Who in America as a "mycologist and ichthyologist" who had discovered "many species . . . of fungi, a number of which have been named in his honor, because of edible or poisonous importance."

83 *Difficulties building the station*: Rensler, Ph.D. dissertation. A typical cable from his secretary told him "The gable looks like hell," to which he replied, "Tear the damn thing off."

83 *Brinkley remained at the stern*: Minnie Brinkley memoir fragment, JRB papers, KSHS.

Chapter 15

84 The story of Miss Lyons's hoax is based on coverage in the Escanaba Daily Press, the Associated Press, the New York Times, Time magazine, and Fishbein, An Autobiography.

Chapter 16

89 *"You accused me of selling"*: *Kansas City Star,* May 8, 1930.

90 Governor Davis blocking extradition: Carson, *Roguish World.*

90 *Rose Sedlacek:* Letter from Mrs. Ruth Sedlacek Woodyard to Minnie Brinkley, April 23, 1976, JRB papers, KSHS. "KFKB, the fourth commercial station in the country, would quickly become first in the nation in terms of listener interest because of the programming genius of John Brinkley" (Lee, *Bizarre Careers*).

Chapter 17

91 *Johann Burckardt Mencken:* For more, see de Francesco, *The Power of the Charlatan.*

91 *drama critic George Jean Nathan:* The waspish Nathan was said to be the model for Addison deWitt in the movie *All About Eve.*

92 *"hypothetical physical agony"*: Angoff, *The World of George Jean Nathan.* See also Hobson, *Mencken: A Life.* Mencken's medical moments weren't all depressing. Writing to Fishbein on September 13, 1924: "I was 44 yesterday: the beginning of menopause. Perhaps it is only a coincidence that the incision in my foot, in healing, takes the form of the female pudenda. There is even a clitoris. . . . The stitches are out, the edges seem to be holding, I am off crutches, and there is no pain. To God be all the glory!" (MF papers, U. of Chi).

93 *"Dear Mr. Mencken, We are sending"*: Fishbein letter to Mencken, April 7, 1922, MF papers, U. of Chi.

93 *One of its articles was entitled:* "Gland Treatment Spreads in America," *New York Times,* May 8, 1925.

93 Dr. Bailey on Harry Thaw: *New York Times,* April 25, 1924. George Bernard Shaw theorized that Oscar Wilde, too, had been led astray by a glandular anomaly.

94 *end of introspective poetry: New York Times,* April 19, 1926, and April 20, 1926.

95 *"[W]e go with expectation"*: *The Idler,* vol. 18, August 12, 1758.

96 For *Pearson's* attack on MF, see "The Sinister Trail of the Medical Trust" by Dr. Andrew A. Gour, *Pearson's Magazine,* June 1924.

96 *"our fun department"*: Snider, draft of Fishbein profile, MF papers, U. of Chi.

Chapter 18

97 *"Watch your prostate for signs"*: Carson, *Roguish World.*

97 *"Note the difference between the stallion"*: Lee, *Bizarre Careers.*

98 *"the most pretentious broadcasting program ever presented"*: Fowler and Crawford, *Border Radio.* For more on 1920s radio programming, see Rensler, Ph.D. dissertation.

99 "*inconceivable that we should allow*": Thomas H. White, "United States Early Radio History," http://earlyradiohistory.us.

99 "*a stench in the nostrils of the gods of the ionosphere*": Quoted in DeForest's obituary, *Time* magazine, July 7, 1963.

99 "*the man who . . . radio as an advertising medium*": Chase, *Sound and Fury.*

99 "*to which most businessmen were blind*": Young, *Medical Messiahs.* Much of the material in this chapter on the rise of radio advertising is drawn from Young and from Chase.

102 "*You could go in there and sit*": Juhnke, *Quacks and Crusaders.*

Chapter 19

103 *Pasteur Institute's emergency monkey farm: New York Times,* January 11, 1925, and January 25, 1925.

103 *from which he increasingly drew his clientele:* Presumably some of these sophisticates enjoyed the Monkey Gland cocktail, made of gin, orange juice, grenadine, and absinthe.

103 *wrapped the monkey glands:* McGrady, *The Youth Doctors.*

104 "*out of the cage*": Friedman, *A Mind of Its Own.*

104 "*The horse is in very good condition*": *New York Times,* December 21, 1923.

104 "*Voronoff told me*": Liardet rhapsodizes at length in *New York Times,* October 7, 1922.

105 Death of Alfred Wilson: Wyndham, "Versemaking and Love-making."

105 "*very satisfied with the result*": Address given at the 12th Annual Conference of the Society for the Scientific Study of Sex, November 1, 1969.

106 "*high-grade person[s]*": A 1926 exhibit sponsored by the American Eugenics movement flashed a light every sixteen seconds to indicate the birth of another citizen, and every seven and a half minutes to indicate the birth of another "high-grade person."

107 "*We have learned*": *New York Times,* February 27, 1927.

107 "*I have far too much respect*": Thorek, *A Surgeon's World.* As a scientist, he deserves much credit in retrospect; he was the only major gland researcher who did not find what he was hoping for.

Chapter 20

108 Chubb flyer: MF papers, U. of Chi.

110 "*We saw Jack Dempsey box*": Marjorie Clavey and Barbara Fishbein Freidell, "Tribute to Morris Fishbein, M.D.," *Medical Communications,* 1977.

111 "*the American Fishbein Association*": Snider, draft of Morris Fishbein profile, MF papers, U. of Chi.

111 *Reasonable minds might differ:* Columnist O. O. McIntyre spoke for the resistance: "Ziegfeld glorifies the American girl, but Morris Fishbein glorifies Morris Fishbein."

111 Mencken stocks up: Teachout, *The Skeptic.*

112 *"The scene of the little German band":* Fishbein letter to Mencken, January 21, 1925, MF papers, U. of Chi.

112 *"[T]here is a shrewd Jew in him":* Mencken diary, December 16, 1943.

Chapter 21

113 Brinkley's visit to Pavia: Carson, *Roguish World.*

114 *"Preaches Fundamentalism":* New *York Evening Journal,* September 11, 1926.

116 *Andy Whitebeck:* Carson, *Roguish World.*

117 *Pavia degree: Kansas City Star,* May 13, 1930.

117 *the degree was personally:* Rensler, Ph.D. dissertation.

Chapter 22

118 Death of Debs: Fishbein, *Fads and Quackery in Healing.*

119 Ekblon episode: *Kansas City Star,* May 11, 1930.

120 Homback episode: *Kansas City Star,* May 18, 1930.

Chapter 23

123 *Brinkley Pharmaceutical Association:* Lee, *Bizarre Careers.*

123 *"Prescription No. 7":* Private circular to druggists of the Brinkley Pharmaceutical Association, undated, JRB papers, KSHS.

Chapter 24

125 Zahner's odyssey is based primarily on reporting in the *Kansas City Star,* especially July 17, 1930, and March 20, 1931.

127 *"She scared me":* Carson, *Roguish World.*

Chapter 25

128 *Dr. H. W. Gilley: Kansas City Star,* especially May 2, 1930.

129 *"It is not in the hope": Kansas City Star,* May 2, 1930.

130 Garvin's letter to Fishbein: February 28, 1930, MF papers, U. of Chi.

130 *"There is nothing the medical profession":* JRB papers, KSHS.

130 *$14,000 a week:* Carson, *Roguish World.*

132 *"treating dangerous afflictions by air": Kansas City Star,* May 7, 1930.

132 *"These M.D.'s are a stinking":* Juhnke, *Quacks and Crusaders.*

132 Baker's stage magic and oil painting by mail: Ibid.

134 *"Tell me frankly":* Fishbein, *An Autobiography.*

Chapter 26

135 *"the most daring and the most dangerous"*: Lee, *Bizarre Careers*.

135 *"The Federal Radio Commission"*: "The Brinkley and Baker Quackeries," *JAMA*, vol. 94, April 19, 1930.

135 *"This scrap on us"*: Broadcast as reported by the *Kansas City Star*, April 11, 1930.

136 *"while some gestures"*: *Topeka Daily State Journal*, April 17, 1930.

Chapter 27

138 *"Mr. Baker had better not come down"*: Fowler and Crawford, *Border Radio*.

139 *"lurid incident"*: "The Baker Ballyhoo," *JAMA*, April 26, 1930.

139 *"up against the strongest"*: Lee, *Bizarre Careers*.

139 *"[I]t could build up"*: W. C. Clugston, *Rascals in Democracy*.

140 Maddox charges: Associated Press, July 17, 1930.

140 *The next day the* Star *published*: The first itemized (though incomplete) listing of clinic deaths appeared in the *Kansas City Star*, May 11, 1930.

Chapter 28

141 goon squad: *Kansas City Star*, May 8, 1930.

141 *"male secretary and fixer"*: Carson, *Roguish World*.

142 *"a regular machine gun of oratory"*: *Kansas City Star*, May 8, 1930.

143 *"KTNT is to be taken off the air"*: Fowler and Crawford, *Border Radio*.

143 he hosted a thrill-packed festival: Juhnke, *Quacks and Crusaders*.

Chapter 29

143 Descriptions of Brinkley's FRC hearing are based on coverage by the *Topeka Daily Capital*, the *Kansas City Star*, the *Kansas City Times*, and the *Washington Post*, among others.

147 *"think of three ways"*: *Smoky Mountain News*, July 31, 2002.

147 *"I suggest you have"*: Chase, *Sound and Fury*.

147 *"I am informed by a friend"*: As transcribed and reported by the *Kansas City Times*, June 16, 1930.

Chapter 30

149 Descriptions of this hearing are taken from transcript of *J. F. Hassig and the State of Kansas v. John R. Brinkley*, 1930, and from coverage of the hearing in the *Junction City Union*, the *Kansas City Star*, and the *Kansas City Times*, among others.

149 *"a spirited exchange of personalities"*: Lee, *Bizarre Careers*.

152 *"absolutely impossible"*: Dr. Thomas Orr, as quoted in Branyan, "Medical Charlatanism."

Chapter 31

155 *"campaign of vindictiveness"*: *Wichita Beacon,* September 21, 1930. See also *Wichita Eagle,* same date.

156 *"In abolition, prohibition"*: Menninger, "Bleeding Kansans," in Averill, *What Kansas Means to Me.*

157 *"two-thirds of a grape crop"*: *Topeka Daily Capital,* September 12, 1930.

157 *to wrap his arms around his father's leg:* A variation on this bit had Johnny Boy running up with papers in his hand.

158 *"from 6:45 in the morning"*: *New York Times,* November 2, 1930.

159 *a midday rally:* Coverage in the *Kansas City Star,* the *Junction City Union,* the *Wichita Beacon,* and the *Topeka Daily Capital.*

160 *"mink and sealskin"*: *Wichita Eagle,* October 29, 1930.

160 *"Garden of Gethsemane"*: Carson, *Roguish World.*

161 *"people's psychologist"*: *Kansas City Kansan,* November 4, 1930.

162 *three counties in Oklahoma:* Carson, *Roguish World;* Mehling, *Scandalous Scamps.*

163 *"there were sufficient votes"*: F. Schruben, *Harry H. Woodring Speaks,* Los Angeles, 1963

163 *Pappy O'Daniel in Texas, everybody:* "His extensive use of the radio . . . his reliance on an airplane for campaign travel, and his inimitable showmanship through ballyhoo rallies revolutionized campaigning in the Sunflower State and the nation" (Lee, *Bizarre Careers*).

Chapter 32

164 *XED, aka "The Voice of Two Republics"*: See "Pioneer Border Blaster: XED," valleystar.com.

165 *Al Scharff in Mexico:* Roark, *The Coin of Contraband.*

165 *commercial bandwidths:* Chase, *Sound and Fury.*

166 *"the only radio Del Rio had seen"*: Braudaway, *Del Rio: Queen City of the Rio Grande.*

166 *Told on a tour that he would need:* Fowler and Crawford, *Border Radio.*

167 *"Whenever he took his favorite pose"*: "Charles Curtis," www.senate.gov.

168 *Maybe he could save his career:* *Collier's,* January 16, 1932.

168 *"The transmitter room was the classic"*: "The Best Darn Story of the Whole 20th Century," www.ominous-valve.com.

168 *XER Gala Week:* Carson, *Roguish World.*

Chapter 33

170 *suicide rate was rising:* Ward, "The Medical Antitrust Case of 1938–1943."

170 *Some men lucky enough:* Allen, *Since Yesterday.*

170 Voronoff and Walska's beauty shop: *New York Times,* April 13, 1927.

171 *"a race of supermen":* New York Times, January 30, 1927; March 17, 1927; September 12, 1927.

171 *"a more complicated physique":* New York Times, May 24, 1928.

171 *"experiments of Professor J. P. Heymans":* New York Times, August 24, 1929.

171 *it was the afterlife that mattered: New York Times,* June 20, 1927.

171 *"might almost be called":* New York Times, April 14, 1927.

172 *"The A.M.A. actually has no legal":* Fishbein writing in *Medical World News,* as quoted by the *New York Times,* February 25, 1973.

173 Henry Junius Schireson et al.: Fishbein, *An Autobiography;* Armstrong and Armstrong, *The Great American Medicine Show.*

173 *"[O]n at least four occasions":* Schwager, "Homage to Morris Fishbein."

173 *"An old eclectic physician":* Fishbein to Mencken, February 26, 1931, MF papers, U. of Chi.

173 *Christian Science healer:* Fishbein, *An Autobiography.*

174 *But the law in those days:* L.N.H., "The First Recorded Murder Conviction of a Medical Quack."

Chapter 34

175 Snake and cave art: See *Texas Monthly* articles by Thompson and Schwartz.

175 *"We played near the station":* Fowler and Crawford, *Border Radio.*

176 XER's international reach: Zwonitzer and Hirshberg, *Will You Miss Me When I'm Gone?*

176 *In later years Russian spies:* Lee, *Bizarre Careers.*

177 *"Hillbilly Hollywood":* Zwonitzer and Hirshberg, *Will You Miss Me When I'm Gone?*

177 *Rose Dawn:* For more on Rose Dawn, see Fowler and Crawford, *Border Radio.*

178 *John the Baptist doll:* Lee, *Bizarre Careers.*

178 Birth of AM radio: "The Best Darn Story of the Whole 20th Century," www.ominous-valve.com.

Chapter 35

179 *"a slugfest like Jack Benny":* Fowler and Crawford, *Border Radio.*

179 *formed a baseball team:* The Spooks, as they were called, were a formidable club, defeating among others the XEPN Whizbangers.

180 *Cowboy evangelist Dallas Turner:* Braudaway, *Del Rio: Queen City of the Rio Grande.*

180 *"Preachers fought off Satan"*: Fowler and Crawford, *Border Radio*.
181 *"by magical arts"*: "National Junta of Quacks," *El Siglo de Torreon*, summer 1932, MF papers, U. of Chi.
181 *"Dr. and Mrs. Brinkley have helped you"*: Form letter, JRB papers, KSHS.
181 *"Highway Safety"*: Carson, *Roguish World;* Fowler and Crawford, *Border Radio*.
181 *"I'm on top of the world"*: *Topeka Daily Capital*, August 2, 1931.

Chapter 36

182 *burned their wheat*: Brendon, *The Dark Valley*.
182 *"an easy mark"*: Fowler and Crawford, *Border Radio*.
182 Brinkley's correspondence with clairvoyants: JRB papers, KSHS.
185 *"extended executive clemency"*: Juhnke, *Quacks and Crusaders*.
185 *"What I want, Dewey"*: JRB papers, KSHS.
185 *"I just realized"*: Schlecta, master's thesis; Juhnke, *Quacks and Crusaders*. The "sound truck" that accompanied Huey Long in his 1930 Louisiana senatorial campaign amplified his voice live.
186 Brinkley in Emporia: "A Crowd Hears Brinkley," *Emporia Gazette*, August 27, 1932.
187 *"Save Kansas!"*: William Allen White, as quoted in *New York Times*, October 2, 1932.
187 Crawford and McCoy: From McCoy's reports, JRB papers, KSHS.
188 *"Do you realize"*: JRB papers, KSHS.

Chapter 37

190 *"This shocked me"*: Edward Bernays, *Biography of an Idea* (Simon and Schuster, 1965).
191 *"ice period of senility"*: *New York Times*, March 21, 1934.
191 *"against his will"*: Gilman, *Making the Body Beautiful*.
192 *eating coal*: For more on the so-called coal hormone, see *New York Times*, July 2, 1933.
193 *"electrical transcription"*: Fowler and Crawford, *Border Radio;* Mendoza, *A Family Autobiography*.
194 *"[Brinkley] has an arresting and highly magnetic"*: Letter from American consul in Piedras Negras, Mexico, to secretary of state, November 20, 1933.
195 *"If your heart goes out"*: Form letter, November 29, 1933, JRB papers, KSHS.

Chapter 38

196 *"I received absolutely"*: Letters are from MF papers, U of Chi.
196 *"I know you are hard up"*: Form letter, August 14, 1934.

197 *If "Senator [Thomas] Sterling of South Dakota"*: Lee, *Bizarre Careers.*
197 Seizure of the Villa Acuna station: Carson, *Roguish World.*
198 *Follow-ups:* Brinkley's virtuosic use of the mail is most completely explored in Rensler, Ph.D. dissertation.
199 *"I've found that when folks"*: Chase, *Sound and Fury.*
199 *E. E. Cooper: Kansas City Star,* May 11, 1930.
199 *"My dear friends"*: Mehling, *Scandalous Scamps.*
199 *$12 million:* Handbook of Texas Online; also Carson, *Roguish World.*
199 *timber, citrus groves, and real estate:* Along the way the doctor even acquired a gravestone company—a way, some thought, for him to make extra money on his less successful cases.
199 *near his boyhood home:* "I asked him for a contribution for the college library once," said Lillian Buchanan, librarian of a college in North Carolina near where Brinkley grew up, "and he promptly sent me 50 copies of his autobiography."
200 *"Till Gabriel blows his trumpet"*: Fowler and Crawford, *Border Radio.*
200 *Huey Long reportedly:* Ibid.
200 The Prostate Gland Warmer, Recto Rotor, and much more can be found on the inexhaustible website of the Museum of Questionable Medical Devices ("the largest collection of medical chicanery and mayhem ever assembled under one roof").
201 *"the finest automobiles, the finest homes"*: Carson, *Roguish World.*
201 *"What more do you want, folks?"*: Fowler and Crawford, *Border Radio.*
201 *Clement Wood:* Wood later wrote the authorized biography of Norman Baker.
202 *promotional film:* Fowler and Crawford, *Border Radio;* Lee, *Bizarre Careers.*

Chapter 39

203 *embroidered with the doctor's name:* Carson, *Roguish World.*
203 *gold buttons and a sword:* Lee, *Bizarre Careers.*
203 *"A trusty who killed three women"*: School report by John Brinkley Jr., JRB papers, KSHS.
204 *"I'd go out to the country club"*: Lee, *Bizarre Careers.*
204 *rented them his yacht:* Fishbein, "The Last Great Quack."
204 *In Halifax the ship was seized: Reno (Nevada) Evening Gazette,* July 5, 1935.
204 *Liverpool, Nova Scotia:* For a detailed description of the fishing scene off Nova Scotia, by Brinkley's close competitor, see Terry Mort, *Zane Grey on Fishing.*
205 *At 788 pounds, it surpassed:* Fowler and Crawford, *Border Radio.*

Chapter 40

206 *"so real that she seemed"*: New York Times, December 4, 1935.

206 *"largely in the effect on the mind"*: Ibid.

206 Yeats and Steinach: For detailed discussions, see Wyndham, "Verse-making and Lovemaking"; Ellmann, "W. B. Yeats's Second Puberty."

207 *"Tickling in back of throat"*: Teachout, *The Skeptic.*

Chapter 41

208 *"sort of a giant golf"*: Associated Press, April 15, 1941.

208 Greenhouse, grounds, and animals: Carson, *Roguish World.*

209 *"How he would fret"*: Fowler and Crawford, *Border Radio.*

209 Brinkley's household treasures: For a meticulous inventory, see JRB papers, KSHS.

209 *cathedral-style, state-of-the-art*: The massive pipe organ was Brinkley's pride and joy. His voluminous correspondence with the Reuter Organ Company regarding custom-made changes taxed even the patience of the fawning company president. JRB papers, KSHS.

210 *"For a poor boy"*: Carson, *Roguish World.*

210 *"He was completely lacking"*: Zina Worley to Gerald Carson, Carson papers, KSHS.

210 *His generous financial contributions*: JRB papers, KSHS.

Chapter 42

211 Brinkley party: *Del Rio Press*, April 23 1937; Lee, *Bizarre Careers.*

211 *with Morris Fishbein on the cover*: Time magazine, June 21, 1937.

212 *Along with the beauty*: Thurber, "La Grande Ville de Plaisir."

213 *Hitler broke out the buckets and brooms*: Wolfe, *You Can't Go Home Again.*

213 Descriptions of the *Normandie*: Braynard, *Picture History of the Normandie;* Foucart, *Normandie: Queen of the Seas.*

214 hemorrhoids and tonsillectomy: Carson, *Roguish World.*

214 *"The doctor worshiped Johnny"*: Unidentified newspaper clipping, MB papers, WMM.

215 Justin and Johnny Boy: Justin Fishbein, author interview.

215 *"Do you know who my boss is?"*: From the testimony of Lowell Brown, *Brinkley* v. *Fishbein,* 1939.

215 Brinkley and Fishbein on deck: Carson, *Roguish World.*

Chapter 43

217 *"Paul Muni, who owes Warners"*: Chicago Herald-Examiner, March 31, 1938.

218 *tiny swastikas*: Lee, *Bizarre Careers.*

219 Atkins, Jennings, et al.: Zwonitzer and Hirshberg, *Will You Miss Me When I'm Gone?*

219 Carter Family material derived chiefly from Zwonitzer and Hirshberg, ibid.; PBS, *American Experience,* "Will the Circle Be Unbroken?"

220 Hadacol: Janette Carter, author interview.

221 *Janette remembered Anita:* Janette Carter, author interview.

Chapter 44

222 Brinkley and Middlebrook: Marinacci, "Getting America's Goat"; Lee, *Bizarre Careers.*

222 *"He was trying to rob":* Zwonitzer and Hirshberg, *Will You Miss Me When I'm Gone?*

223 *he took over the Crescent Hotel:* Fowler and Crawford, *Border Radio;* Juhnke, *Quacks and Crusaders.*

223 *But Middlebrook declined:* Carson, *Roguish World.*

Chapter 45

224 *"the biggest bunch of grafters":* Personal letter from JRB to Mrs. C. E. Lusk, April 20, 1933, AMA files.

225 *"for the notions of every nit wit":* Ward, "The Medical Antitrust Case of 1938–1943."

226 *"scurvy liars"* and other quotes: Bode, *New Mencken Letters,* August 16, 1938.

Chapter 46

227 *"Whenever A.P. wanted to say":* Fowler and Crawford, *Border Radio.*

228 Brinkley letter to his attorneys: MB papers, WMM.

Chapter 47

231 John R. Brinkley *v.* Morris Fishbein: To Gerald Carson, Brinkley's lawsuit was "a supreme effort, a kind of Pickett's Charge."

232 *embossed on it in thirteen places:* Fowler and Crawford, *Border Radio.*

233 Letters to Fishbein: MF papers, U. of Chi.

Chapter 48

235 Trial coverage: *Del Rio Evening News, San Angelo Standard-Times, San Antonio Express,* Associated Press.

235 Clinton Giddings Brown's background: Brown, *You May Take the Witness.*

236 *"and that is where I seen this article"*: Most of the testimony that follows is quoted verbatim. Some fragments have been compressed for clarity.

237 *"a little man with a little goatee"*: Fishbein, *An Autobiography.*

238 *"I consider Dr. Brinkley"*: *San Angelo Evening Standard*, March 23, 1939.

240 *"The whole bunch of them"*: Brown, *You May Take the Witness.*

Chapter 49

242 Fishbein's testimony: Transcript, *Brinkley* v. *Fishbein*. Morris Fishbein defended his book, *Modern Medical Home Remedies*, by saying it was intended for spot help or emergencies, not as a substitute for a doctor's care. Nevertheless, even some supporters viewed it as a kissing cousin of *Medical Question Box*.

Chapter 50

248 Brinkley's testimony: Transcript, *Brinkley* v. *Fishbein*.

Chapter 51

253 Brinkley's testimony: Transcript, *Brinkley* v. *Fishbein*. The "weight or volume" exchange is described in Carson, *Roguish World.*

Chapter 52

263 *"appalling denunciation"*: Oscar Wilde, *De Profundis.*

263 *"I want to win"*: Carson, *Roguish World.*

265 *"If we can beat him"*: Lee, *Bizarre Careers.*

265 *"[H]ow on earth"*: MF papers, U. of Chi.

265 *"Leslie Banks is the scientist"*: *New York Times,* April 9, 1939.

Chapter 53

266 *dressed as a slave:* Ronald L. F. Davis, "Popular Art and Racism," jimcrowhistory.org; Ira Katznelson, *When Affirmative Action Was White* (W. W. Norton, 2005).

266 Description of the *GWTW* premiere: *New York Times,* December 16, 1939.

267 *"has rendered our client"*: Carl E. Langston to Morris Fishbein, August 23, 1939, MF papers, U of Chi.

268 *"Dear Friend"*: Form letter, March 1, 1940, JRB papers, KSHS.

268 *"where full confidence"*: Lee, *Bizarre Careers*. Brinkley went so far as to send out a form letter: "Announcing the location of the Brinkley Hospital, Inc., in the beautiful Roswell Hotel in sunny Del Rio, Texas, near the silvery Rio Grande and romantic Old Mexico." But he was too impoverished and harassed to follow through.

268 For more on Brinkley and the Dilley Aircraft School adventure, see Carson, *Roguish World;* Better Business Bureau Bulletin, December 9, 1940.

269 *"Nassau is beautiful"*: JRB papers, KSHS.

269 *"I never had any books"*: Carson, *Roguish World.*

269 *six horses:* Arkansas Democrat, March 24, 1941. See also "Brinkley Relates Tale of Vanishing Rio Grande Empire," *Wichita Eagle,* March 25, 1941.

270 *"I am bankrupt"*: Lee, *Bizarre Careers.*

270 *"Honey, It seems my heart"*: JRB papers, KSHS.

Chapter 54

271 *"When Dr. Brinkley"*: Minnie Brinkley memoir fragment, JRB papers, KSHS.

271 *"The American Medical Association"*: JRB papers, KSHS.

271 *"I guess there isn't any danger"*: Carson, *Roguish World.*

271 Brinkley's and Minnie's begging letters: JRB papers, KSHS.

272 *carbolic acid, and water:* The formula was revealed in September 1931, during testimony in Baker's unsuccessful suit against the AMA.

273 *"We are being tried"*: JRB papers, KSHS.

273 *"What a little tinkering"*: "The Mystery That Was Brinkley," *Emporia Gazette,* n.d., AMA files.

273 *"The centuries to come"*: Lee, *Bizarre Careers.*

273 *"I knowed he was bilking me"*: "The Subtle Knife," NYPRESS.com.

Epilogue

274 *"a murderer without a license"*: Ambrose Bierce, *The Devil's Dictionary.*

274 *go to jail for murdering a patient:* L.N.H., "The First Recorded Conviction of a Medical Quack."

275 *"Hank Snow, Ernest Tubb"*: Fowler and Crawford, *Border Radio.* Elvis Presley, however, was barred.

275 *"They became very popular in Mexico"*: Fowler and Crawford, *Border Radio.*

276 *Bob Smith of Brooklyn:* The Wolfman Jack material is taken primarily from his autobiography, *Have Mercy! Confessions of the Original Rock 'n' Roll Animal.*

276 *"an all-American music"*: New York Times, May 24, 1987.

277 *rough signs:* For more on modern-day "health" clinics in Mexico, see Ron Rosenbaum, "Starchild Abraham: His Trip to Tijuana for Chemo-Refusal," *New York Observer,* August 7, 2006.

279 *"glowing skin, increased muscle mass"*: Hoberman, *Testosterone Dreams.*

279 *cancer and premature death:* Much of the surrounding material is drawn from the *New York Times:* "Anti-Aging: Potion or Poison?" April 12, 1998; "Quest for Infinite Youth Raises Hopes and Cash," July 22, 2003; "Growth Hormone: The Secret of Youth or a Cautionary Tale?" April 11, 2006. See also Haber, "Life Extension and History," and Hall, *Merchants of Immortality.*

280 *resveratrol:* "Yes, Red Wine Holds Answer. Check Dosage," *New York Times,* November 2, 2006.

280 *"I wish it were possible":* Benjamin Franklin, letter to Jacques Dubourg, April 1773.

280 *"forty-five years ahead of his time":* Topeka Capital-Journal, April 22, 1976.

281 *"Do you remember":* ZZ Top, *Fandango,* 1975.

Selected Bibliography

Books

Allen, Frederick Lewis. *Since Yesterday.* Harper & Bros., 1940.

Anderson, Ann. *Snake Oil, Hustlers and Hambones.* McFarland & Co., 2000.

Angoff, Charles, ed. *The World of George Jean Nathan.* Alfred A. Knopf, 1952.

Armstrong, D., and E. Armstrong. *The Great American Medicine Show.* Prentice-Hall, 1991.

Atherton, Gertrude. *Black Oxen.* Boni and Liveright, 1923.

Averill, Thomas Fox, ed. *What Kansas Means to Me.* University of Kansas Press, 1995.

Bealle, Morris. *Medical Mussolini.* Columbia, 1939.

Bernays, Edward. *Crystallizing Public Opinion.* Boni and Liveright, 1923.

———. *Propaganda.* Horace Liveright, 1928.

Bode, Carl. *The New Mencken Letters.* Dial, 1977.

Braudaway, Douglas. *Del Rio: Queen City of the Rio Grande.* Arcadia, 2002.

Braynard, Frank O. *Picture History of the Normandie.* Dover, 1987.

Brendon, Piers. *The Dark Valley.* Alfred A. Knopf, 2000.

Brinkley, J. R. *The Brinkley Operation.* Sydney B. Flower, 1922.

Brown, Clinton Giddings. *You May Take the Witness.* University of Texas Press, 1955.

Bufwack, Mary A., and Robert K. Oermann. *Finding Her Voice: Women in Country Music, 1800–2000.* Vanderbilt University Press, 2003.

Bullough, Vern L. *Science in the Bedroom: A History of Sex Research.* Basic Books, 1994.

Capote, Truman. *In Cold Blood.* Random House, 1965.

Carson, Gerald. *The Roguish World of Dr. Brinkley.* Rinehart, 1960.

Casey, Robert J. *More Interesting People.* Bobbs-Merrill, 1947.

Chase, Francis, Jr. *Sound and Fury.* Harper & Bros., 1942.

Clugston, W. G. *Rascals in Democracy.* Richard R. Smith, 1940.

Corners, George F. *Rejuvenation: How Steinach Makes People Young.* Thomas Seltzer, 1923.

Cramp, Arthur J. *Nostrums and Quackery.* Chicago, 1936.

David, Charles A. *Greenville of Old.* Historic Greenville Foundation, c. 1998.

de Francesco, Grete. *The Power of the Charlatan.* Yale University Press, 1939.

deKruif, Paul. *The Sweeping Wind.* Harcourt Brace, 1962.

Dougan, John. *Memphis.* Arcadia, 2003.

Drury, John. *Dining in Chicago.* John Day Co., 1931.

Dye, Robert W. *Memphis (Then and Now).* Arcadia, 2005.

Fishbein, Morris. *An Autobiography.* Doubleday, 1969.

———. *Fads and Quackery in Healing.* Blue Ribbon, 1932.

———. *The New Medical Follies.* Boni and Liveright, 1925.

Foucart, Bruno. *Normandie: Queen of the Seas.* Vendome Press, 1985.

Fowler, Gene. *Mystic Healers and Medicine Shows.* University of New Mexico Press, 2001.

Fowler, Gene, and Bill Crawford. *Border Radio.* Texas Monthly Press, 1987.

Friedman, David M. *A Mind of Its Own.* Free Press, 2001.

Gardner, Martin. *In the Name of Science.* Putnam, 1952.

Gilman, Sander L. *Making the Body Beautiful.* Princeton University Press, 1999.

Gottlieb, R. *Thinking Big: The Story of the Los Angeles Times, Its Publishers and Their Influence on Southern California.* Putnam, 1977.

Haire, Norman. *Rejuvenation.* Macmillan, 1925.

Hale, Annie Riley. *These Cults.* National Health Foundation, 1926.

Hall, Ben. *The Best Remaining Seats.* Clarkson N. Potter, 1961.

Hall, Stephen S. *Merchants of Immortality.* Houghton Mifflin, 2003.

Hallinan, Joseph. *Going Up the River: Travels in a Prison Nation.* Random House, 2003.

Hansen, Harry. *Midwest Portraits.* Harcourt Brace, 1923.

Hecht, Ben. *Child of the Century.* Simon & Schuster, 1954.

Hering, Daniel. *Foibles and Fallacies of Science.* D. Van Nostrand, 1924.

Hoberman, John. *Testosterone Dreams: Rejuvenation, Aphrodisia, Doping.* University of California Press, 2005.

Hobson, Fred. *Mencken: A Life.* Random House, 1994.

Holbrook, Stewart. *The Golden Age of Quackery.* Macmillan, 1959.

Jastrow, Joseph, ed. *The Story of Human Error.* D. Appleton-Century, 1936.

Juhnke, Eric S. *Quacks and Crusaders: The Fabulous Careers of John Brinkley, Norman Baker, and Harry Hoxsey.* University Press of Kansas, 2002.

Lee, R. Alton. *The Bizarre Careers of John R. Brinkley.* University Press of Kentucky, 2002.

Lewis, Grace Hegger. *With Love from Gracie.* Harcourt Brace, 1955.

Lewis, Lloyd. *It Takes All Kinds.* Harcourt Brace, 1947.

Lewis, Lloyd, and Henry Justin Smith. *Chicago: The History of Its Reputation*. Harcourt Brace, 1929.

Lingeman, Richard. *Sinclair Lewis: Rebel from Main Street*. Random House, 2002.

Longstreet, Stephen. *Chicago*. David McKay Co., 1973.

MacDougall, Curtis D. *Hoaxes*. Macmillan, 1940.

Mackay, Charles. *Extraordinary Popular Delusions and the Madness of Crowds*. Bonanza Books, 1981.

Malone, Bill C. *Country Music, U.S.A*. University of Texas Press, 1968.

Manchester, William. *Disturber of the Peace*. Harper & Bros., 1951.

McCoy, Bob. *Quack! Tales of Medical Fraud from the Museum of Questionable Medical Devices*. Santa Monica Press, 2000.

McDougal, Dennis. *Privileged Son: Otis Chandler and the Rise and Fall of the L.A. Times*. Perseus Books, 1990.

McGrady, Patrick M., Jr. *The Youth Doctors*. Coward-McCann, 1968.

McNulty, Elizabeth. *Chicago Then and Now*. Thunder Bay Press, 2000.

Mehling, Harold. *Scandalous Scamps*. Henry Holt, 1959.

Mencken, H. L. *My Life as Author and Editor*. Alfred A. Knopf, 1993.

———. *The Diary of H. L. Mencken*, edited by Charles A. Fecher. Alfred A. Knopf, 1989.

Mencken, Johann Burckhardt. *The Charlatanry of the Learned*. Alfred A. Knopf, 1937.

Mendoza, Lydia. *A Family Autobiography*. Arte Publico Press, 1993.

Miner, Craig. *Kansas: The History of the Sunflower State*. University Press of Kansas, 2002.

Mitgang, Herbert, ed. *Letters of Carl Sandburg*. Harcourt Brace, 1988.

Montana, Patsy, and Jane Frost. *Patsy Montana: The Cowboy's Sweetheart*. McFarland, 2002.

Morrow, Mayo. *Los Angeles*. Alfred A. Knopf, 1933.

Mort, Terry, ed. *Zane Grey on Fishing*. Lyons Press, 2003.

Porter, Roy. *Quacks: Fakers and Charlatans in Medicine*. Tempus Publishing, 2004.

Rascoe, Burton. *Before I Forget*. Doubleday, 1937.

Roark, Garland. *The Coin of Contraband*. Doubleday, 1964.

Sandburg, Carl. *Chicago Poems*. Henry Holt, 1916.

Sawyers, Julie Skinner. *Chicago Sketches*. Wild Onion Books, 1995.

Schorer, Mark. *Sinclair Lewis*. McGraw-Hill, 1961.

Schruben, Francis W. *Kansas in Turmoil, 1930–1936*. University of Missouri Press, 1969.

Sigafoos, Robert. *From Cotton Row to Beale Street*. Memphis State University, 1980.

Steiger, Brad. *Bizarre Crime*. Penguin, 1992.

Steinach, Eugen. *Sex and Life: Forty Years of Biological and Medical Experiments*. 1940; reprint, McGrath, 1970.

Sullivan, Mark. *Our Times*. Vols. 5 and 6. Scribners, 1926–1935.

Teachout, Terry. *The Skeptic: A Life of H. L. Mencken*. HarperCollins, 2002.

Thorek, Max. *A Surgeon's World*. J. B. Lippincott, 1943.

———. *Camera Art*. J. B. Lippincott, 1947.

Time-Life. *This Fabulous Century, 1910–1920*. Time-Life Books, 1969.

———. *This Fabulous Century, 1920–1930*. Time-Life Books, 1969.

Trimmer, Eric J. *Rejuvenation: The History of an Idea: The Search for the Fountain of Youth*. London, 1967.

Ulin, David L., ed. *Writing Los Angeles*. Library of America, 2002.

Voronoff, Serge. *Life*. Dutton, 1920.

White, William Allen. *Selected Letters*, edited by Walter Johnson. Henry Holt, 1947.

Wolfe, Thomas. *You Can't Go Home Again*. Harper & Bros., 1940.

Wolfman Jack, with Byron Laursen. *Have Mercy! Confessions of the Original Rock 'n' Roll Animal*. Warner Books, 1995.

Wood, Clement. *Life of a Man*. Goshorn Publishing, 1934.

WPA. *Texas, A Guide to the Lone Star State*. American Guide Series, 1940.

Young, John Harvey. *The Medical Messiahs*. Princeton University Press, 1967.

———. *Toadstool Millionaires*. Princeton University Press, 1961.

Zwonitzer, Mark, with Charles Hirshberg. *Will You Miss Me When I'm Gone?* Simon & Schuster, 2002.

Magazines and Newspapers

...temporary coverage in *Kansas City Star, Kansas City Times, Kansas City Journal-Post, Topeka Daily Capital, Topeka Daily State Journal, Wichita Beacon, Wichita Eagle, Emporia Gazette, Del Rio (Texas) Evening News, Greenville (South Carolina) Daily News, Chicago Tribune, Chicago Herald and Examiner, Escanaba (Michigan) Daily Press, Los Angeles Times, New York Times, New York Evening Journal, Washington Post*, and others.

Articles

"Ballad of A. P. Carter." *Life* magazine, December 1991.

Ballou, Dr. W. H. "Gland Transplantation Is Link in Chain of Scientific Progress." *Life and Letters*. Girard, Kansas, n.d.

Brammer, Bill. "Salvation Worries? Prostate Trouble?" *Texas Monthly*, March 1973.

Branyan, Helen B. "Medical Charlatanism: The Goat Gland Wizard of Milford, Kansas." *Journal of Popular Culture*, vol. 25, Summer 1991.

Bryk, William. "The Subtle Knife." NYPRESS.com, May 27, 2003.

Ellmann, Richard. "W. B. Yeats's Second Puberty: A Lecture Delivered at the Library of Congress on April 2, 1984." Library of Congress, 1985.

Fishbein, M. "John R. Brinkley—Quack." *JAMA,* vol. 90, February 14, 1928.

———. "Modern Medical Charlatans." *Hygeia,* vol. 16, January–February 1938.

———. "The Last Great Quack." *Coronet,* April 1945.

Haber, Carol. "Life Extension and History: The Continual Search for the Fountain of Youth." *Journal of Gerontology,* vol. 59A, 2004.

Herman, John R., M.D. "Rejuvenation: Brown-Sequard to Brinkley." *New York State Journal of Medicine,* November 1982.

Hogeland, William. "The Inventors of Commercial Country Music." *New York Times,* August 1, 2004.

Korry, Edward M. "Is This Man Keeping the Pope Alive?" *Look,* December 10, 1957.

Leland, John. "High on a Hilltop with Music All Around." *New York Times,* August 8, 2002.

L.N.H. "The First Recorded Conviction of a Medical Quack." *Connecticut Medicine,* July 1964.

Marinacci, Michael. "Getting America's Goat," pw2.netcom.com.

Oudshoorn, Nelly. "Endocrinologists and the Conceptualization of Sex." *Journal of the History of Biology,* Summer 1990.

Prebel, Julie. "Engineering Womanhood: The Politics of Rejuvenation in Gertrude Atherton's *Black Oxen.*" *American Literature,* June 2004.

Rosenbaum, Ron. "Starchild Abraham: His Trip to Tijuana for Chemo-Refusal." *New York Observer,* August 7, 2006.

Schulteiss, D., J. Denil, and U. Jonas. "Rejuvenation in the Early 20th Century." *Andrologia,* vol. 29, 1997.

Schwager, Edie, ed. "Homage to Morris Fishbein." *Medical Communications,* vol. 5, no. 4, 1977.

Schwartz, Eileen. "Prehistory Lesson." *Texas Monthly,* June 2002.

Shah, J. "Erectile Dysfunction Through the Ages." *BJU International,* September 2002.

Shaw, Jonathan. "The Aging Enigma." *Harvard Magazine,* September–October 2005.

Thompson, Helen. "Snakes Alive!" *Texas Monthly,* July 1993.

Thurber, James. "La Grande Ville de Plaisir." *New Yorker,* January 29, 1938.

Time magazine. Morris Fishbein cover story, June 21, 1937.

Ward, Patricia Spain. "The Medical Antitrust Case of 1938–1943." *American Studies,* Fall 1989.

Wardlaw, Frank. "The Goat-Gland Man." *Southwest Review,* Spring 1981.

Wright, Willard Huntington. "Los Angeles—the Chemically Pure." *Smart Set,* March 1913.

Wyndham, Diana. "Versemaking and Lovemaking—W. B. Yeats' 'Strange Second Puberty': Norman Haire and the Steinach Rejuvenation Operation." *Journal of History of the Behavioral Sciences,* Winter 2003.

Archives

John R. Brinkley papers, Kansas State Historical Society, Topeka, Kansas.

Minnie Brinkley papers, Whitehead Memorial Museum, Del Rio, Texas.

Gerald Carson papers, KSHS, Topeka, Kansas.

Morris Fishbein papers, Special Collections Research Center, University of Chicago.

Fishbein-Mencken correspondence: MF papers, University of Chicago and Special Collections, New York Public Library.

Academic Works

Rensler, Ansel Harlan. "The impact of John R. Brinkley on broadcasting in the United States." Ph.D. dissertation, Northwestern University, 1958.

Schlecta, Don B. "Dr. John R. Brinkley: A Kansas Phenomenon." Master's thesis, Kansas State College, Hays, 1952.

Radio Archives

Recordings of Brinkley broadcasts, Radio Archive of the University of Memphis and the Aaron Mintz Vintage Radio and Television Archive.

Online Sources

Museum of Questionable Medical Devices, NYPRESS.com, sniggle.net, museumofhoaxes.com, and others.

Index